"This great resource offers the wisdom of experts on the creative process, who share their own challenges in completing creative projects. With clarity and kindness, they explore the characteristic challenges that creatives face and present individualized strategies for completion. This guidance on how to remove blocks and fuel creativity is a major contribution to the coaching field."

Leia Francisco, *author of* Writing Through Transitions

"This book is a treasure-trove! Packed with ideas and strategies to help creatives with the never-ending challenges of being creative, it provides great tips on how to stay the course, experience the flow and complete your projects."

Sandra Marinella, *author of* The Story You Need to Tell

"What creative person has not struggled with seeing a creative project through to completion? Roadblocks, detours, distractions and psychological upheavals are all par for the course. This book serves as a candle in the dark for those who dare to create and can use the support, insight and wisdom of fellow travelers on the path."

Eric Teplitz, *writer, musician, coach and*
host of The Person You Want to Be *podcast*

"If you are someone who starts things but has a hard time finishing them, you are not alone. Don't let your creative dreams go unfulfilled! Let this book inspire and guide you with what it takes to complete your creative work! You will find practical ideas, tips and strategies from others who know how to get things done. If you are a creativity coach, you will find many tools and approaches for helping your clients complete their creative pursuits. I strongly recommend this book to anyone who wants to get what matters done."

Rebecca Kochenderfer, *founder, Journaling.com*

"*The Coach's Guide to Completing Creative Work* provides readers with excellent suggestions and approaches to meeting one's creative goals. Discussed are commitment, organization, routines, motivation and much more. I highly recommend this book to anyone needing that extra push to get to the finish line."

Merle R. Saferstein, *author of* Living and Leaving My Legacy, Vol. 1

T0383394

"In the midst of a writing project, this book has helped me more firmly grasp the slippery and ornery nature of the creative process. Wherever you are in your creative journey, Maisel, Monk and colleagues offer practical insights for meeting the challenges of completion. I promise that this book will fortify your creative practice!"

Ruth Folit, *writer*

"*The Coach's Guide to Completing Creative Work* demystifies the difficulty of finishing creative work. Both obstructions and solutions are laid out clearly, simply, personally and usefully. In an organized and enjoyable manner, a variety of articulate creative people help all of us in the fight against the inner and outer blockages to creative success."

Beth Jacobs, *author of* A Buddhist Journal

"I've long struggled to make the shift into structure and organization that completion requires. But thanks to this beautifully crafted and emotionally nourishing collection of wisdom coaching, I have strategies galore for my upcoming end stage."

Kathleen Adams, *Center for Journal Therapy, author of*
Journal to the Self *and* Expressive Writing: Foundations of Practice

"The collaborative writing and editing team of Eric Maisel and Lynda Monk has done it again! If you're an artist or writer who's bumped into the stumbling blocks of procrastination, perfectionism, or other such limiting practices, *The Coach's Guide to Completing Creative Work* is a creative lifesaver. With more than forty chapters written by coaches, artists and writers, this guide is a cornucopia of ideas, suggestions, advice and encouragement for creatives of all stripes. This is a book that I need, that I'll use and that I can't wait to share with others on the creative path."

Judy Reeves, *author of* A Writer's Book of Days *and*
Wild Women, Wild Voices

The Coach's Guide to Completing Creative Work

This book brings together 38 creativity coaches from around the world to offer coaches, therapists, creatives and clients accessible and practical tools to get their creative work done.

Curated by two leading creativity coaches, these chapters seek to help coaches and clients alike tackle common challenges that all creatives face when finishing a project. Chapters cover topics such as procrastination, failure, accountability, perfectionism, mindfulness, the importance of support, perseverance and more, with each section finishing with tips for both clients and coaches that can be used in sessions. Filled with rich case studies and true stories from creativity coaches throughout, this book addresses the current issues of our times, such as the distractions of social media, remote working and the effects of the COVID-19 pandemic.

Applicable to a range of creative disciplines, this book is essential reading for coaches, therapists and their creative clients looking to complete their creative work efficiently and effectively.

Eric Maisel is the author of 50+ books, among them *Inside Creativity Coaching: 40+ Inspiring Case Studies from Around the World, The Creativity Workbook for Coaches and Creatives: 50+ Inspiring Exercises from Creativity Coaches Worldwide* and *Transformational Journaling for Coaches, Therapists and Clients: A Complete Guide to the Benefits of Personal Writing*, all published by Routledge.

Lynda Monk is the director of the International Association for Journal Writing (IAJW.org) and co-editor of *Transformational Journaling for Coaches, Therapists and Clients: A Complete Guide to the Benefits of Personal Writing*. She is co-author of *Writing Alone Together: Journaling in a Circle of Women for Creativity, Compassion and Connection*. She is passionate about the transformational and healing power of writing.

The Coach's Guide to Completing Creative Work

Top Tips for Working with Procrastination, Perfectionism and More

EDITED BY ERIC MAISEL AND LYNDA MONK

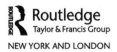

NEW YORK AND LONDON

Designed cover image: jc_design © Getty Images

First published 2023
by Routledge
605 Third Avenue, New York, NY 10158

and by Routledge
4 Park Square, Milton Park, Abingdon, Oxon, OX14 4RN

Routledge is an imprint of the Taylor & Francis Group, an informa business

ISBN: 978-1-032-39779-5 (hbk)
ISBN: 978-1-032-39778-8 (pbk)
ISBN: 978-1-003-35134-4 (ebk)

DOI: 10.4324/9781003351344

Typeset in Avenir and Dante
by Apex CoVantage, LLC

To my husband, Peter, an artist,
and our two sons, Jackson and Jesse,
and our beloved golden retriever, Sadie – *love has no end*.
It is completed moment by moment.

To Ann, 45 years into this adventure.

Contents

Co-Editor's Introduction

Lynda Monk

Through the years, we have all likely heard a well-meaning person advise us to stop procrastinating and get this or that done. Just the other day, I suggested to my teenage son that he should really get his overdue homework done before he goes out fishing. He went fishing anyways, of course he did! We all go fishing, literally or metaphorically from time to time, instead of getting the other important things done. Even when you think to yourself, "I really should get this done" or "I really want to finish writing my book," still, you might avoid it. Despite our best intentions to get something done once and for all, time passes, and our creative dreams can go unrealized.

This book brings together creativity coaches, artists and writers to unpack what it takes to successfully complete creative work. While we naturally will not complete everything we start, if we can complete MORE of what we start, we benefit and so do others. Completion is the essential ingredient for *living* our creative dreams and not just *thinking* about them.

> "Creative projects in your head help no one."
>
> —Sam Horn

My Story

I have started and completed many things in my life, including three university degrees, various projects, books, businesses and a first marriage. I have written or co-written over 100 training programs, teaching manuals, online courses and articles. I have co-authored and co-edited four published books. I have facilitated training workshops with many thousands of participants over the years. I have parented two sons. This does not have a completion, thankfully, but is worthy of mentioning as there is an element of completion in so many moments of transition throughout their childhoods, so many milestones that mark completion of one phase of growth to another. This is true of our creative work as well. We move through phases, stages and milestones to completion.

I have also NOT completed things – creative projects I have started, articles, blog posts, new products that get partially created and never see the finish line. And then there are the various book projects that I have started, where I've made folders, written the table of contents, created book proposals and early chapters, but not gotten to the finish line. All these potentially fabulous endeavors just sit incomplete in my computer or, with older projects, on my office shelf in printed form.

Why Is That?

Firstly, as a creative person and you can probably relate, I get A LOT of ideas. For example, I can get ten new journal product ideas a day for our journaling store, usually before I have finished my first cup of coffee. Some I never act on, some I take a little action on, some I take a lot of action on and yet still don't complete. Some are designed, done and benefitting the people who buy them.

Some projects are bigger than others. For example, I have been working on my memoir on and off – mostly off – with the exception of short bursts of momentum during writing retreats where I immerse myself in the project. It is not only a larger project defined by length but also a deeper project based on the emotional presence it takes to process and share my story as an adoptee. It takes more courage to write because it is personal, makes me feel vulnerable and involves the people I love the most. It is easy to procrastinate, to avoid it and not to finish it. It is also painful not to complete something that I know I am here to give birth to in this lifetime. I am working on it.

Some creations are more interesting to me. I find the projects that I truly love and find interesting are the ones that most often make it to the finish line. Passion and a sense of purpose are good motivating forces that support completion.

Some projects have deadlines and paydays. When I am working on projects that clients are paying me to create – for example, developing workshops, training programs, course curricula, keynotes and presentations – they *always* make it to completion.

Pause and reflect: What things inspire and motivate you to complete your creative work? What things get in the way of completing it?

Working Alone and Working with Others

I have worked for over two decades as a self-employed entrepreneur, where completing creative projects has been the core of my work in one form or another. I have mostly worked independently and I have at times worked with others.

There is great value in collaborative work when it comes to completion. Collaboration can also slow things down as it takes more discussion and planning time and, well . . . collaboration. When it comes to completion and all that leads up to it, things like momentum and deadlines, even self-imposed ones, can be successfully achieved working with others. I have had buddy systems, mastermind partners, co-working times with colleagues who are also creating things, writing groups I have been part of in the past and business partners. These have all advanced my creative pursuits in some useful way. There are the synergy of ideas, mutual support, the enjoyment of working with others, accountability and many other benefits to collaboration, including how it can support us to complete things.

I have completed many things working alone and I have completed many things working in collaboration. Some people have a strong preference for one way or the other for getting things done.

Pause and reflect: It is good to ask yourself what commitments you keep more often – the ones you make to others or the ones you make to yourself? Another thing to consider is how self-motivated you are and if you can put structures, routines and habits in place each day that support you to complete your creative work.

Stages of Creation

We all know that there are various stages in any creative project. There is the starting, progressing and completing. This does not always, or ever, happen in a linear process and I have rarely experienced a straight line through any creative pursuit, although there are necessary steps to completion. Regardless of how the path unfolds, there are some very real things we must face and DO to stand at the finish line with our creative work successfully completed. This book presents you with many ideas, tips and strategies intended to help you complete the creative work that you are here to do.

I believe the creative sparks that come to us are given to us for a reason. Certain things are meant to come through us in this lifetime. I believe our lives are enriched and we make a difference with our work when we follow these callings, these sparks and turn them into the creations they are meant to become – a book, a painting, a piece of music, a course, a screenplay, a photograph. Let's make our mark. Let's make a difference with our art. Let's listen to the call of our souls. Let's get it done.

We are living in complex times that require us to do our creative work. Beauty heals. Art matters. Creativity is not just something we *do* but it is part of *who* we are. Completion is a way of honoring who we are and of affirming the meaning in our lives.

> *Don't bend; don't water it down; don't try to make it logical; don't edit your own soul according to the fashion. Rather, follow your most intense obsessions mercilessly.*
>
> Franz Kafka

My co-editor, Eric Maisel, is letting Chapter 1 serve as his introduction to the book's themes. That chapter comes next. We truly hope this book supports and inspires you to complete *your* creative work.

Why Completing Creative Work Is So Darn Hard

1

Eric Maisel

Many creatives have no particular trouble starting projects but lots of trouble finishing them. Why is finishing a novel, a memoir, a song, or a painting so problematic for so many artists? Here are 12 reasons, framed from the point of view of a painter. I'm sure that you'll be able to easily translate these points to the medium in which you work.

1. The Painting-in-Progress Doesn't Match Your Original Vision for the Piece

Very often, an artist "sees" her painting before it is painted – sees it in all its beauty, grandeur and excellence – and then, as she paints, the "real" painting in front of her doesn't match the brilliance and perfection of her original vision. Disappointed, she loses motivation to complete her creative project and either white-knuckles her way to the end or, in fact, doesn't complete it.

One solution? Understand that your real paintings will be different from your imagined paintings. Maybe every so often they will be identical – but most of the time they won't. The reality of process pretty much guarantees that the work you are doing will "go its own way" and will become the thing it will become, not some remembered or idealized version of itself. Maturely accept that any feelings you may harbor for the idealized or remembered version of your piece should not prevent you from accepting – and appreciating – the real version in front of you.

DOI: 10.4324/9781003351344-1

2. The Hard Bits Won't Come

Even if you successfully complete 99% of your work of art, if 1% remains that still isn't working or that doesn't satisfy you, then that work of art remains incomplete in your own estimation.

What do artists try to do in this situation?

- Some have the happy experience of returning to that 1% and the solution suddenly presents itself.
- Some decide to "keep fussing with" the troubled area, maybe finally bringing it to completion or maybe making a mess of the whole thing.
- Some decide to call the work of art "finished for now" and put it out in the world with that nagging 1% still lacking.
- Some decide to step away from the work of art for a period of time, in the hope that when they come back to it, either they will know what to do or the problem will have vanished of its own accord.
- Some abandon the work altogether and number it among those creative efforts that didn't quite pan out.

There is no perfect solution to this natural dilemma. It is simply the case that sometimes a part of the thing we are working on isn't coming around. Because this is true so often, many of our creative efforts are held hostage to this problem. When your work of art is 99% done and 1% remains recalcitrant and intractable, what tactics will you employ to get to the end?

3. The Fear That This Is Your Best Idea

Let's say that you've been working for months on a large, complicated narrative painting. You've figured out how to take a mythological subject and put it into modern dress and you're both proud of and excited by your idea.

Naturally enough, your brain has organized itself around this idea, is focused on this painting and isn't allowing neurons to fly off and think about other paintings and other ideas. This natural phenomenon of being focused has a shadow side, however: it can make you believe not only that you don't currently have another good idea but also that you *won't* have another good idea . . . ever.

Your brain can fool you into thinking that this excellent idea is the last excellent idea you'll ever have. You can get weighed down by the feeling that since no other idea will ever come to you, you had better nurse this one so as to have something to work on and to put off what you feel will be a terrible moment of reckoning when, with this painting done, you face the void and discover that you have nothing left to say.

The antidote is simply to say "No!" to this half-conscious thought that this is your last good idea ever. Even if no next idea is currently present, that is no reason to presume that an excellent idea won't percolate up when the time is right, after this painting is completed. Remind yourself of the following: that it is wonderful that you are enjoying your current idea but that it will likewise be wonderful to encounter your next idea, which is bound to become available once your brain has completed its thinking on this painting.

4. The Appraising Will Have to Begin

While you're working on a piece, you can keep saying to yourself, "Yes, maybe it isn't wonderful yet, but by the end it will be!" You hold out the carrot that your further efforts will transform the work into something you really love. But once you say it is complete, then you actually have to appraise it and decide if it is or isn't excellent or even any good.

Because we want to put off that moment of reckoning, we are inclined to say, "Well, let me do just a little more." Out of conscious awareness, we may know that there isn't really anything more to do and that maybe doing more will actually harm the work. But still, we continue to tinker because we don't want to have to confront the question, "Okay, since I am calling it done, is it any good?"

The answer: accept that appraising is coming. That appraising isn't the end of the world. You may be wonderfully surprised; you may be pleasantly surprised; and, yes, you may be disappointed and even demoralized, but whatever the outcome, it isn't the end of the world. You can chalk your effort up to process, part of your apprenticeship and just the natural fact that only a percentage of your work will prove to be excellent and move right on.

Try not to continue working on a project just because you fear the moment of appraisal. Fear that moment less and you will finish things much more easily, quickly and regularly!

5. Lack of a "Completion Checklist"

If you're building a house and you're approaching the end of the project, you create a punch list of last things that have to get done: spot painting, putting in a last switch plate or light fixture and so on. When you've completed everything on your punch list, you can be pretty certain that you are done. Yes, you still have to look around to see if you've missed anything. But you can feel pretty confident that, because you got everything checked off your punch list, you are probably really done or very close to done.

By contrast, a visual artist likely has no such checklist or punch list, would probably never dream of creating one and, even if the concept popped into his head, would probably have no idea what to put on such a list. And yet it can prove helpful to consider this checklist idea and see if it might serve you.

Let's say you're a super-realist painter whose current painting comprises a tabletop, a bowl of apples, a vase of flowers and a collection of tabletop mirrors filled with various reflections of the apples, the flowers and the other mirrors. You could conceivably make a list that included each apple, each flower, each mirror and so on and as you completed each element of the painting, you might check that element off.

One painter might find such an approach too mechanical, analytical, or even nonsensical, but another painter might find such an approach useful. Whether or not such an approach seems useful to you, the main idea remains a very important one: because visual artists typically do not have checklists or punch lists that help them complete projects, they must find their own ways of knowing when a painting is done. If a punch list might work for you, excellent! And if it makes no sense to you, then you are obliged to find other ways to know when your painting is done.

6. Lingering Doubts

It's very hard for most people not to doubt themselves sometimes – especially when it comes time to say that one of their creative projects is successfully completed. An artist who finishes a painting may almost instantly have his mind throw up a doubt or some other unhelpful thought of the following sort:

- "Maybe I should do more because there's always more to do."
- "Maybe I'm done, but am I really 100% certain about that cast shadow over there on the right?"
- "Maybe I'm done, but it doesn't exactly look like what I had in mind for this painting."
- "Maybe I'm done, but have I really answered all those objections raised by that gallery owner in London about whether I'm successfully cultivating a unique painting style?"

- "Maybe I'm done, but a painting is never really done, so how can I say that I'm done?"
- "Maybe I'm done, but wouldn't just a little work there and a little work there improve it?"
- "Maybe I'm done, but . . ."

If one of these is the habitual way your mind plays tricks on you and keeps you from completing things in a timely and appropriate way, it is your job to get a grip on your mind. When you hear yourself doubting yourself in one of these unfortunate ways, exclaim, "No! I know that thought! It doesn't serve me and I don't want it! No, you darn thought, no!"

Who but you is in a position to put doubts of these sorts to rest? If you are plagued by doubts that are the equivalent of you experiencing some ambient anxiety and, as a consequence, pestering yourself unnecessarily, you must silence those doubts instantly!

7. Ongoing Conflicts About What and How Much to Reveal

All artists expose themselves in their art. One artist may expose his sexual fantasies or his sexual obsessions. Another artist may expose her rages and resentments. A third may expose an unpopular belief or violate some cultural rule or norm. An abstract artist may fear that his audience will suppose that he can't really draw, even though he can and by painting abstractly expose himself to suppressed or overt ridicule. Even the most "innocent" sort of work, in which, for example, the subject matter is a bowl of apples or a vase of roses, is an exposure of sorts, perhaps, in a conflicted artist's mind, exposing his lack of innovation or imagination.

All art says something about the artist – and an artist may be conflicted about whether she likes what her art says about her or what it reveals about her. The easiest way to deal with this conflict is to not complete things: then no one will ever see your art and no exposure or ridicule is possible. Many artists fail to complete their works of art because they are in an inner battle about whether or not they are happy with what their art reveals about them.

The answer is to bring this conflict into conscious awareness and deal with it. Decide one way or the other whether you are willing to reveal your sexual fantasies, your simmering rage, or your disagreements with your society. Say out loud, "I am not worried in the slightest that I'll be charged with not being able to draw," or "I don't care at all what people infer about my imagination – or lack of imagination – because I want to paint apples and roses." Decide your position on these issues and then stand behind your decision! If you stay on the fence, the likelihood is great that your work will not get done.

8. Difficulty Knowing If and When Your Work of Art Is Complete

A minimalist, Zen-influenced painting might be done after just a few strokes. A narrative painting might have a cast of dozens of characters and require countless strokes. Is the former less complete than the latter because it is minimalist and so much of the canvas remains white and bare? No, of course not. Each must be considered complete according to its own criteria for completion, its own aesthetics and its own lights. But how confusing this can become! We look at our work in progress and simply can't tell if it is "done already" or "needs more work."

Many artists have the deep, visceral feeling that their work is done early on in the process and their continued work on it actually weakens the effect. How odd! Because "completion" is necessarily a subjective assessment and not an objective assessment and because we may experience multiple contradictory feelings of this sort, we must ultimately simply make a decision, one that is more like a guess and a surrendering than a calculation or a foregone conclusion. If we do not regularly surrender in this way and announce that a given work is done, then it isn't and never will be. It will always remain unfinished. An artist's central task is to engage in this special poignant surrendering – as uncertain as he may still feel as he makes his decision.

9. Fear of Losing Your Happy Place

You're doing a series of red paintings. All that red is making you happy, buoyant and joyful. You have it in your mind that you will do a blue series next and while that makes sense to you intellectually and aesthetically, it doesn't move your heart much. All this red feels wonderful to you; the coming blue feels a little cool, verging on cold. So as to keep this loving feeling alive, you decide just out of conscious awareness not to finish these red paintings. You just want a little more time with them!

Or maybe you're painting a complicated cityscape and you simply love the city that you're translating and transcribing. You love its shapes, its resonances, its history and its shadows – you love everything about it. So you decide, just out of conscious awareness, to keep adding to the scene because you don't want to leave it. In this way, you keep at this painting far longer than you really need to – maybe even to the point of ruining it with too many objects and too much attention.

The mantra to remember is that more love is available after this project is finished. Maybe the blue series will, indeed, prove cooler than the red series – but maybe the yellow series that comes after the blue series will bring back fiery passion. Maybe this cityscape is, indeed, enthralling – but the next one might enthrall you, too. You may have to mourn leaving this happy place, but leave it you must – for the sake of completing your works of art and for the sake of your new loves to come.

10. Not Being Ready for the Process to Start All Over Again

Some artists can't wait to finish their current work of art and begin their next one. They feel perpetually eager to begin, see with each new canvas or each unused ball of clay a new problem to solve or a new beautiful object to make and hold completing their current work of art as the necessary stepping stone to their next creative adventure.

At least as many artists, however, have the opposite reaction. They find starting each new work of art something of a trial and even a little traumatic. At the moment of needing to begin, they pester themselves with questions like "Do I have another good idea in me?" and "Am I really working in the right style?" and "Will this be just another one of my paintings that no one wants?" Because beginning is so painful a process for them, they prefer to keep working on their current project, even if it is done or could readily be completed, rather than face the unpleasant reality of another blank canvas.

If you are in this second group, you need to improve and maybe even heal your relationship to starting. You don't want starting to feel so terrible that it prevents you from completing! Try to answer the following question and then implement your answer: "If starting is a miserable point in the process for me, what can I do to make it less miserable?"

11. Not Being Ready to Start Showing and Experience All That Potential Criticism, Silence and Rejection

While you are working on your current piece, you can say to anyone who inquires about it and asks to see it, "Sorry, it's not finished yet." If they beg, you can hold your ground and repeat your message: "Sorry, it disrupts my process if I show things before they're done." But how can you refuse them once you call the work done? What reason can you possibly offer up that doesn't make it clear that you're balking simply because you fear a cruel remark or an indifferent response? Once you affirm that your current work of art is done, you don't really have a leg to stand on if you try to keep it hidden.

Since artists know that they don't have a leg to stand on once they finish their work of art, they contrive a great solution: they don't finish it. They may get "very near" to the end on many paintings but, by virtue of not having completed any of them, achieve their half-conscious goal: they can righteously announce that they have nothing to show yet. In this way, they keep all possible criticism, rejection and negativity at bay.

The better solution is to grow a thicker skin and get easier – much easier – with letting your works of art out into the world. Yes, since every work of art is disliked by someone, it is indeed the case that some negativity is bound to come your way. Accept that; surrender to that truth, finish your work and show it.

12. Not Being Ready to Start Selling and to Experience All That Potential Criticism, Silence and Rejection

Some artists are natural-born salespeople and love the marketplace. Most artists are extremely reluctant salespeople and a sizeable number despise treating their works of art as commodities.

Not only is selling art difficult and often unpalatable; the act of submitting your works of art for sale brings up the specter – and the likelihood, verging on the certainty – that you will be met regularly (and far too often) by silence and indifference on the one hand and criticism and outright rejection on the other.

Few artists want this silence, indifference, criticism and rejection and many artists find such interactions so painful that they avoid them at all costs. One simple way to avoid the painful side of selling art is not to complete your works of art. There are other ways, too – by completing things and then putting them aside and letting them accumulate, by making such limited efforts at marketing that they hardly count as marketing at all, etc. – but, by far, the simplest way and the way chosen by lots of artists, is simply not to complete things.

If you are caught up in this dynamic, try to break this cycle right now. Spending frustrating year after frustrating year not completing your works of art because you loathe or fear the marketplace is a very bad idea. Please try to get easier with the marketplace and decide to brave it. You may not love this idea, but is having three-quarters-finished works of art piling up the happier prospect?

 ## About the Author

Eric Maisel is the author of 50+ books. His recent books include *Why Smart Teens Hurt*, *Redesign Your Mind* and *The Power of Daily Practice*. Among his other books are *Coaching the Artist Within*, *Fearless Creating*, *Rethinking Depression* and *The Van Gogh Blues*. Dr. Maisel writes the *Rethinking Mental Health* blog for *Psychology Today*, with 3,000,000+ views and is the creator and lead editor for the Ethics International Press Critical Psychology and Critical Series. A retired family therapist and active creativity coach, Dr. Maisel's forthcoming books include *The Coach's Way* (New World Library) and *Deconstructing ADHD* (Ethics International Press). Dr. Maisel provides workshops, webinars and keynotes nationally and internationally; trains creativity coaches; and facilitates support groups for writers. You can visit him at www.ericmaisel.com and contact him at ericmaisel@hotmail.com

The Stories We Tell Ourselves

2

Clare Bunting

The energy of finishing a project can be very different from the energy of starting one, don't you think? I'm nearing the final draft manuscript of my current work in progress. I remember the excitement I had when I started, imagining holding the finished book in my hands and the looks on the readers' faces as they turned the pages. But now, fatigue has set in and I wonder when my work will be done. In spite of this, I know there are things I can do to help myself get over the finish line.

So what does it take to finish a creative project? Once your client has created the work, improved their craft and done a few rounds of revision, part of the challenge may be in understanding if they are stalling or if there really is more work to be done.

I imagine you've come across well-meaning artists who have advised you to stick to a schedule. "You can't keep revising forever," they say. "You'll edit the magic out of it." Perhaps you've met others who told you to keep working until you've done all you believe you can with your work. Of course, it's up to your clients to decide which route they believe is going to bring them closer to their desired result.

Is it more important to get the painting in the exhibition sooner rather than later? Is it more important to give the novel a better shot of being published by spending more time developing it? Is it more important to stop messing around with the content so the original ideas stay fresh?

When I'm on my own timeline and I see ways to improve or add more depth to my work, I'll strive to make the changes even if that creates a delay or means that a small amount of the original magic is lost. But I also know there are stories that we all tell ourselves that may keep us stuck.

DOI: 10.4324/9781003351344-2

Take Louise, an imagined writer, who you may have met. Louise lives with her husband and their Labrador, Billie. She works in a bank to pay the bills. She's writing the fifth draft of a psychological crime thriller. In the hopes that she will finally finish her book, Louise visits a creativity coach.

Louise's coach asks, "What's stopping you from finishing the novel?"

"I've got a full-time job," Louise replies. "There just aren't enough hours in the day. I'm often away visiting friends with my husband on weekends, so I can't always manage to write then."

"How much time do you need to finish your book?" the coach asks.

Louise says she might be able to finish her novel if she had seven hours per week for the next four months.

Hearing what Louise has said about not having enough time, the coach asks her to do a time inventory between now and the next session.

When Louise returns a fortnight later, her coach asks, "What did you get from doing the time inventory?"

"That I'm really busy. But I already knew that," Louise says.

"Last session, you said you could finish your book if you had a free seven hours per week for the next four months. Is there anything on your time inventory that you could give up and replace with writing?"

Louise runs through her inventory and confirms she can't give anything up.

Through the conversation, the coach finds out that Louise spends half an hour every morning on social media, something that she doesn't want to give up for four months to finish the book. Louise's reasoning is that this is her time of peace. After some more questions, Louise says that the peace actually comes from the quiet and the cup of tea she drinks while she scrolls through social media. "My husband's alarm hasn't gone off yet and I have half an hour's quiet time just for me."

"If I remove the social media from the process, do you still get peace?" the coach asks.

"I think so," Louise replies.

"And if I reduce the time to five minutes?"

"That's too short," Louise says.

"Eight minutes?"

"Okay."

"Imagine waking up, sipping your tea in bed for eight minutes. Would that give you the peace you need to set you up for the day?"

"Yes," Louise replies.

"So you wake up, have your tea and quiet time for eight minutes. That gives you twenty-two extra minutes every morning. What would you like to do with this extra time?"

"I'd like to write," Louise says. "But I need more than twenty-two minutes to write."

"How many minutes do you need?"

"At least forty-five."

The conversation continues and at the end of the session, Louise says she'll wake up twenty minutes earlier and make her lunch the night before, which gains her a total of fifty minutes every weekday morning to write. She says she'll make up the rest of the time on the weekend.

At the next session, Louise says she's frustrated. She managed to do her new routine three mornings the first week, but the following week, she was back on social media most mornings and she hadn't done any writing over the weekends. She discussed some strategies with her coach, which included buying an alarm clock, leaving her mobile phone in the other room and taking her iPad offline so she couldn't go on social media and visualizing the reader engrossed in her book before she started writing. She also came up with a writing routine for the weekends and a strategy for making up any missed writing hours in the evening to stop the guilt of missing a session getting the better of her.

During the next session, Louise's coach was interested to find out that while Louise had achieved more writing (four hours the first week and three hours the next), she was still resistant. She returned to one of the questions she had asked Louise in the first session: "What's stopping you from finishing this novel?"

"I haven't got enough time," Louise says.

"What's stopping you?" the coach repeats.

"I haven't got enough energy."

"What's stopping you?"

"It's too hard."

"What's stopping you?"

"I'm not good enough."

"What's stopping you?"

"I never finish anything."

"What's stopping you?"

"Writing makes me feel guilty. I should be spending time with my husband."

"What's stopping you?"

"My husband will leave me."

Later, Louise says that she was surprised by her responses. She didn't realize that not feeling good enough and not having enough energy were making her resist getting the work done. What particularly surprised her was her response about her husband. She says it had never crossed her mind that her husband would leave her if she stayed at home to write occasionally instead of socializing with him and their friends. The coach asks Louise what difference knowing this makes to her. Louise says she'll need to think about it.

At the next session, Louise says that feeling guilty for writing instead of spending time with her husband makes her remember her father's behavior toward her mother when she was a child. She says her father used to try to make her mother feel guilty about taking her and her sister to swimming lessons because he had to eat dinner on his own.

"What difference does making this connection make?" her coach asks.

Louise sighs. "I feel lighter. The guilt isn't mine."

After three more months of writing and working through her challenges with her coach, Louise finishes her novel. She has written for at least three mornings out of five and four hours most weekends and she has worked on understanding that she has the time, letting go of feelings of guilt that didn't belong to her and working on her craft until it's the best it can be without sabotaging her progress.

"What's the difference between now and five months ago?" her coach asks.

"Energy," Louise says. "I spend my time and energy writing instead of spending all my time thinking about why I can't write."

 Three Tips for Creatives

1. Do a time inventory for one week to understand how you spend your time. Is there anything you can cut from your routine and replace with creating?
2. Grab a pen and paper and ask yourself 20 times, "What's stopping me from finishing this project?" Look at the list of reasons. Then challenge each one.
3. Think about a time when you finished something successfully. What did you do differently that you aren't doing now? What can you learn from this? What strategies would you like to put in place to help you finish your creative project?

Three Tips for Coaches

1. Ask your clients questions to help them connect with their original passion, purpose and motivation for wanting their work to exist in the world.
2. Find out what stories your clients are telling themselves about why they haven't finished their creative work. Do any themes come up? Perhaps perfectionism is kicking in. Perhaps they're afraid to share their work with the world. Perhaps this isn't the right project for them. Challenge their stories where appropriate.
3. If your clients are interested, help them come up with a plan of how to reach the finish line and what strategies they will put in place to get back on track if they fall behind.

About the Author

Clare Bunting is a coach and EFT practitioner and also writes for kids. She helps people work through challenges and carve out time for their creative work.

Failure Is an Option 3

Dianne Ochiltree

When I first began writing this chapter, I asked colleagues and clients if they'd like to publicly share their stories about a time when something they'd judged negatively as a failure turned out to be a positive success in the end.

Takers? Not a one.

Failure, it seems, is the other f-word we rarely mention in polite conversation. Yet if we are working in the creative arts, we should – because rather than being something to avoid, failure is an integral part of a healthy creative process.

Until we understand this truth at a cellular level, we put our creativity in jeopardy. The fear of failure can stall us and, in the end, become a major obstacle to completing our creative work.

Speaking from experience with my own work and that of my creativity clients, here are four common ways a fear of failure threatens our ability to complete creative work:

1. We create small. We repeat themes or styles or topics that were a "success" in the past. We play it safe rather than creating with courage and curiosity. Our work is stale, boring and not likely to be completed.
2. We're easily distracted from our creative work in progress. If no outside diversions are handy, we create them. We avoid failure one interruption at a time. Sadly, such distractions knock us off track for an hour, a day, a week, or more.
3. We abandon creative projects midstream to start something with more promise of "success," then quickly cast it off for another bright and shiny start. This stop-and-start work pattern creates nothing but an endless cycle of non-completion.
4. In a worst-case scenario, our hidden fear of failure grows so large, we may halt creating anything. We have abandoned not just our many uncompleted projects but our creative souls as well.

DOI: 10.4324/9781003351344-3

All this is a high price to pay for an unreasonable – and many times unconscious – fear.

So, how *do* we combat fear of failure as creators? A good place to start is by understanding some truths behind that f-word.

Truth #1: Failure Is an Essential Tool for Success

We don't learn or discover or create without a so-called "failure" or two along the way.

Thomas Edison's beleaguered attempts to create a light bulb can serve as inspiration for our own creative journeys. As he himself famously said, "I have not failed. I've just found 10,000 ways that won't work."

Like Edison, we must commit ourselves to the long haul, relying on patience and persistence. Any time a "failure" arises as you work, give yourself permission to take a breather – three slow, deep breaths to the count of four – and recommit yourself to opening up to wherever the muse takes you next.

Truth #2: Failure Doesn't Define Us; It Refines Us

Failure is a not just a natural part of the creative process; it is a useful tool for elevating our voices, vision and versatility. Our unique and authentic creative self is refined each time we allow ourselves to "fail" through trial and error, detours and dead ends, sometimes winding up at a creatively satisfying destination in our completed works.

Imagine one of those robotic floor vacuum sweepers in action. It zooms around the room, collecting whatever little bits it encounters in one direction, then swivels around to sweep in another direction, collecting more little bits there. By attacking the mess from every angle – sometimes even backtracking – the sweeper has created a masterpiece of a clean floor.

A healthy creative process proceeds similarly. We explore in one direction, discover something new, file that knowledge away, then go down other creative alleyways, one at a time. Our skills, knowledge and confidence grow when we allow ourselves to create in this manner.

We must expect twists and turns on our creative path. Our "failures" guide us toward creative completion in a sure, if somewhat zigzag way.

Truth #3: Failure Is a Judgment, Not a Fact

Rather than an objective fact, failure is a subjective judgment, often formed by others. We may buy into ideas about failure consciously or unconsciously. But we don't have to! We ourselves are the only ones qualified to define "failure" or "success" in our work. And remember, it serves us well not to judge anything during the creative process itself.

Truth #4: Failure Exists Only Where Expectation Exists

Expectation is the enemy of happiness . . . and creativity. If we go into our creative process expecting a specific outcome in a specific time frame, we open ourselves up to judging our work in progress as either a "failure" or "success." Can you perhaps just be curious about all your discoveries?

Truth #5: If We Treat Failure Kindly, It Will Return That Kindness

We all must rethink the language we use in self-talk as we travel the naturally twisting path of creation. Before our inner critic even gets the chance to chide us for a "failure," we can instead congratulate ourselves for a brave experiment. In addition, we can also be kinder in our evaluations of what we've bumped into along our merry, messy way by asking ourselves positively framed questions, such as "What's working here?" or "What did I just learn from this?" or "What can I try next?" to help us decide what to keep or discard for our next go-round.

I believe that if we can frame failure in a positive light, if we name it and claim it as the valuable mentor and the guide it was always meant to be, we can gather much that supports our creative life.

Truth #6: Failure Isn't Fatal; It Brings Creativity to Life

For years, a fear of failure held me hostage. It still sometimes rears its ugly head! But I've learned that a failure, public or private, is not the end of things. Rather, it is the beginning of something that I wouldn't have discovered otherwise. Failure truly sparks my creative spirit.

Welcoming the necessity of *"failure"* to our creative process turns each detour into an opportunity to grow our technical skills and self-confidence as a creator. It eliminates one more potential obstacle to success at completing our creative projects, too.

Yes, failure *is* an option. And a smart one, at that.

Three Tips for Creatives

1. Manage your expectations. Remember, our work can only be judged a failure or success when we expect a particular outcome. Take a moment to write down any expectations you might have with your work in progress. Then destroy the piece of paper you've put them on. Crumple it and toss it in the trash, rip it to confetti in the document shredder, even burn it to ashes. Poof! Once expectations and fear of failure are released, dive into creating. Chances are you will not only complete that project, but you'll also have fun doing it.

2. Create a failure-friendly mindset. Populate your workspace with reminders of failure's valuable presence in your creative process. Post inspirational quotes on Post-it notes; create and display simple affirmations, such as "Failures are steps to completion," or "When I create, I cannot fail." Weave supportive practices into your workday as well. Light a candle as a signal to the universe that you're ready to let your creative light shine no matter the twists and turns of your process. Sit quietly for a minute of meditation before you set to work, breathing deeply and repeating in your mind an affirmation that resonates with your creative soul, such as "Failure fuels my creative process," or "Failure is my teacher and friend."

3. Fail like a champ. Remember the words of author C. S. Lewis: "Failures, repeated failures, are posts on the road to achievement. One fails forward toward success." See if you can internalize the truth that failure is a necessary step toward creative expansion and completion. Think about past times when you thought you had failed at your creative task. Did you really fail in the end? My guess is you will find lots of personal examples that illustrate the transformative power of allowing mistakes and failures to bring new knowledge and skill into your work.

Three Tips for Coaches

1. Play detective. Ask open-ended questions that will encourage your client to explore negative beliefs hiding behind a fear of failure. Perhaps "Why do you think you've come to a stop?" or "How do you fear you might fail here?" or "Which aspect of this project causes you doubt?" or "What would failure look like to your way of thinking?" will help start a useful discussion. It needn't be a lengthy or complicated conversation – just enough to tag the major block to creative completion. Then ask, "Is this negative self-belief true?" Almost always, the answer is no. A false belief is easier to disbelieve.

2. Encourage and empower. Whatever the suspected underlying cause of fear, you can help your client flip the switch on their relationship to failure. Ask, "What would you do here if you knew you couldn't fail?" After actively listening to the responses, you might give assurances that all these things can be done because happily, there is no such thing as a failure in the creative process. Your assurance that so-called "failures" are nothing more than necessary steps will empower your creative client to complete that work in process with confidence. Ask your client to visualize themself as a young child at play in the sandbox or finger-painting in preschool. There was no fear of failure there, was there? Assure your client that they can be a creative free spirit as a grownup, too.

3. Fill their toolbox. Working together, brainstorm the tools and techniques that will help your client tame the fear of failure when creating. Together, create a menu of habits that support the healthy acceptance of so-called failures and mistakes. This might include affirmations, meditations, breath work, rituals, inspirational quotes, journaling prompts, or daily practices. What seems to resonate with your client? It's important to generate something that works for the individual and to resist "fixing" things in a rote manner.

 ## About the Author

Dianne Ochiltree is a published children's author, writing coach and freelance editor with over 25 years of publishing experience. She helps her clients discover their authentic voices and polish their work until it shines. To learn more, please go to www.dianneochiltree.com.

How Creative Rituals Help Get Things Done

4

LA Bourgeois

Tall grass outside my window turns the early morning light a little green. When I glance up from my keyboard, a laughing Buddha figurine smiles at me. The dog snores on a nearby bed.

Check the clock. Ten minutes until breakfast. I type faster.

As a professional freelance writer, I devote four to six hours each weekday to writing. While my dream of being a writer included capes, a settee for reading and a desk out of a manor from an Agatha Christie novel, the truth of freelance writing is days upon days of me hunched over a laptop. My fingers, hands and arms ache while I find the focus and bravery to continually draft pieces of writing, submit the work and ask for more. I had to build up to this point and my ritual made that happen.

Finding the time for my creative goals was similar to wedging a screwdriver into the tiniest crack to open it up. I discovered that the screwdriver must stay in the crack. If I remove it, that small space slams shut.

That screwdriver is my ritual.

Now, some people might just call this process I'm about to describe a routine. A habit. And it's both those things. For me, naming it a ritual emphasized the process and the importance of my writing.

Rituals Are for Important Things

My writing is important to me. It's my art. It's my creative expression. It's how I delight readers and one way I enable them to create beauty joyfully.

DOI: 10.4324/9781003351344-4

However, I wasn't treating my writing as important. Instead, much of my time was spent on other duties, with my own art as an afterthought. As much as I wanted to build a creative habit, resistance roared whenever I made the attempt.

Then I began thinking of the church services of my youth. How, each Sunday, the service proceeded through the same actions. Here we stood. The candles were lit. At this point, we sang. The songs may have been different and the words of the sermon changed from Sunday to Sunday, but the order of the actions remained the same. The ritual that was maintained – and is still maintained – gave each parishioner a framework on which to express their spirituality.

The framework of a ritual could give me the same opportunity to express my creativity. Plus, by elevating my creative habit to a ritual, I immediately felt the importance of my work increase. That scared me and almost set me back on my heels, but the framework of the ritual helped. The repetition each weekday slowly proved to me that my work was as important as the ritual itself, that what was occurring in that little room where I write was sacred.

Rituals Are About the Process

When we hold our rituals, the rite is the event. They are the thing, in and of themselves. No matter what comes out of the ritual, the ultimate goal is simply to hold it, to be in it, to sing the songs and rejoice and enter into the contemplation and accept the sacredness of the process.

To my mind and muse, a creative habit felt like something that needed to be done to produce the product. And in my perfectionist mindset, my product wasn't good enough. How would I make the product good enough? Only through showing up and engaging in the work. By shifting my goal from the product to the process, I was able to push through my resistance. Performing the ritual, rather than finishing the book, became the goal.

Commit to the Ritual Through Preparation

Each ritual requires some preparation. Candles and matches gathered. Appropriate clothing. Music to be rehearsed. Food prepared.

After settling on the order of my ritual through visualization and testing, I realized that I needed to make room for my ritual by preparing the next workday's lunch the night before. So, as I cleaned up after dinner, I made my lunch and stored it in the refrigerator. That freed up my fifteen minutes of ritual time in the morning. It also meant that each evening before I went to bed, the ritual had already begun, even when I hadn't typed a single word. Each evening, as I made my salad, I committed to performing the ritual the next morning and had that thought as I went to sleep. This commitment made it possible, when I woke the next morning, to follow through and complete my ritual.

How the Ritual Supports Completion

In its final form, my ritual included a physical action that committed me to the work, an intent to do the work and a plan that could be completed on most days. And note the "most" in that last sentence. Just like all of us, I have days when I sleep late and still must get the trash out and clean the litter box. When I had a day job, that meant that my fifteen minutes of writing couldn't happen.

By creating a ritual that emphasized the commitment and the intent to do the work, when those days showed up, I knew I'd still succeed even if no words made it onto the page. That feeling of success brought me back to the ritual the next day, clear of defeating self-judgment. More days than not, I completed my fifteen minutes of writing until I started to feel ready for more.

I began to use that ritual to wedge my day open even further. I increased my work time by just five minutes at first and then in fifteen-minute increments. After several months, I wrote for an hour each morning. And then came the big leap. I winnowed away my time at my day job, going from full time to part time and then to the barest amount of contract work before leaping completely away into this new life of professional writing and coaching.

Rituals can elevate the process of the work, exchanging questioning of the quality for the assuredness of the creative performing their craft.

 Three Tips for Creatives

1. Create a ritual that helps you focus on the process. Every creative has points when they doubt their end product. Will it be good enough? Will the world love it? Can it happen faster? However,

before the end product can be produced, the work must be done. By shifting the focus from the end product to the process, the work can proceed, research done, processes refined, practice maintained. A ritual makes the process important, rather than the end product.

2. A ritual doesn't have to happen every day. At first, I worried about not writing every day. Even though my weekends were filled with necessary errands and rejuvenating for the coming week, if I didn't write every day, would I falter in my goals? Think about it: do people forget to go to church on Sundays? As a lapsed churchgoer, I can attest that you never really forget. Even today, I will wake up on a Sunday and snuggle up with a novel, my wife and my dog, relieved that I don't have anywhere to be at 11:00 a.m. If churchgoers could have a ritual that kept them coming back once every seven days, I could have a ritual that took time off over the weekends and that has worked for me. If you feel like you must do your work every day, please soften that to every day-ish so that when you inevitably have your creative practice derailed by life, you still can have a feeling of success at the end of the week.

3. The ritual starts with the preparations. Taking an action to prepare for the ritual begins the commitment to perform the ritual. You are deciding to make it easier to do the ritual than not and this decision propels you toward your creative practice.

Three Tips for Coaches

1. Use a ritual with a client who struggles to focus on the process. When I saw my practice as a ritual, I began to see my power in the process. I could show up and perform my ritual practice each weekday and be a success at that, even when I doubted my talent and craft. This shifted my idea of success from an end product that found appreciation in others' eyes to simply showing up with the intent to write. That hit of success each time I showed up kept me returning to the work.

2. Use a ritual with a client to help them see the importance of their creative work. Many creatives are perfectionists like me and therefore reject doing the necessary work to complete a project because it isn't perfect or worthy. Using a ritual to perform that work elevates the practice to the sacred duty of the creative and begins to break

down the resistance to seeing their work and, eventually, their product as sacred, even when it isn't perfect. However, elevating the work to this level of importance can trigger feelings of inadequacy in the client. This danger point must be moved through with gentle encouragement and recommendations to persist.

3. Help the client see that the preparation for the ritual begins the commitment to doing it. By preparing for the ritual, the client makes the space for the ritual to occur and makes the commitment to perform the ritual. Encourage the client to regard their preparations as part of their sacred duty to perform the ritual, just like washing the tools for church service, such as communion cups and special garments, is seen as holy.

 ## About the Author

LA (as in tra-la-la) Bourgeois is a Kaizen-Muse–certified creativity coach and freelance writer who encourages you to embrace joy as you manifest your creative goals. Her creativity writing is informed by Eric Maisel, Twyla Tharp and Jill Badonsky and uses Badonsky's Kaizen-Muse creativity tools. Battle resistance, procrastination and overwhelm with her at your side, gently encouraging with humor and heart. Discover more at her website, labourgeois.biz.

The Joy of Completion   5

Clare Thorbes

When it comes to completion, the ability to self-coach is vital for creatives and creativity coaches. With some shifts in attitude and a few practical techniques, you can learn to love the process of completing your creative projects.

Attitude

Like many of the artists I knew (even the successful ones), I used to dread showing my work. Facing an audience was an excruciating experience. I used to cringe, wondering what caustic comments would come my way during an exhibition. I think it kept my productivity low. The somewhat unconscious negative self-talk went something like this: if I don't finish paintings, I don't have to risk public ridicule. The resulting snail's pace of completion ensured that it took me a lot longer than necessary to develop as a painter and start to get positive feedback instead of dismissive remarks.

One of the mental shifts that finally helped me was realizing how differently each person sees a given painting or experiences any of the arts. People have a range of opinions, but what matters much more is how artists feel about their own work. If I can honestly say that I've pushed myself to do the best I can at a given stage of my artistic career, then my vulnerability to imagined and real negative comments is greatly reduced. That's my completion standard and it makes outside judgment almost irrelevant. I've also replaced thoughts like "I have so much left to do, I'm not sure I can face it!" to "All I have left to do is . . ." and "One more session and it's done."

Another attitude shift occurred as I started working on my current series of paintings. I thought I'd need at least 20 paintings for a proper solo show. Although I had good momentum, I got so busy with other obligations that

DOI: 10.4324/9781003351344-5

I made myself sick with stress and drove myself crazy with negative self-talk: Am I going to make my self-imposed deadline? Will I have to postpone my show? If I do, will I lose that precious momentum?

Then I asked myself how many pieces I actually needed. Deciding that 12 or 14 paintings would be enough took a lot of the pressure off. I relaxed and began to really enjoy completing the paintings at a slower pace. I decided not to let the numbers bother me anymore. Now my attitude is: How many paintings will be enough? As many as I get done.

Techniques

Regular Mini Showings

Showing my work before it was finished was something I would never have dreamed of doing earlier in my painting life. One day, I invited a friend into my studio to look at some unfinished pieces because I wanted to share my love of making art with her. I knew that even if she didn't like the pieces, she would be kind. Instead, she said, "I don't know what I'm looking at." I realized how much timidity exists on the viewer's side as well. I got the chance to explain what I was doing and she was eager to learn how the raw material became a painting. We never got around to assessing the work; it just didn't seem important.

When I started on my latest series, I regularly showed the pieces in progress to two or three close friends in my new city. It always gave me a boost because I knew they had seen a lot of art over the years and would understand that they were viewing unfinished pieces. This quick sharing of cell phone snapshots of the work proved to be a powerful habit and I lost my remaining fear of showing. I got a real kick out of presenting my latest efforts as they evolved and I felt I had my friends' moral support. That gave me the momentum to keep completing new pieces. I even gained enough confidence from these mini-exhibitions to admit when I took a wrong turn with a piece or didn't quite capture the effect I wanted.

Visualization

By imagining an exhibition of the series, I changed reluctance into pleasurable anticipation as I mentally worked out where I'd show, whom I'd invite and how I'd display the pieces for maximum impact. My vision included a room full of enthusiastic viewers. I take that imagined scenario into the studio each day so that I feel I'm surrounded by supportive fans who are nudging me along.

Tracking

I created a table in Word, listing the paintings I wanted to complete, the status of each one and next steps. Instead of losing time to indecision at the start of each painting session, I now check my list and ask myself which one feels easiest or is closest to completion. The tracking system helps me quickly choose which painting to work on that day. This way, pieces are completed on a fairly consistent basis. It also keeps me upbeat as I work. I know I'm moving steadily closer to the solo exhibition and the evidence that I'm getting there is in my tracking system and in the completed pieces on the walls around me. That, in turn, motivates me to seize small moments in the day to make bits of progress on some of the paintings.

Celebrate

When I complete a painting, I make a point of celebrating. I treat completion as the victory it is and I whoop and sing and dance around the room on a wave of euphoria!

 Three Tips for Creatives

Just as it's possible to convert your inner critic from your most stubborn adversary to your most useful ally, you can develop a powerful inner stance toward presenting your creations to the world. Try these tips to overcome self-doubt and the fear of exhibiting or performing.

1. Mini-exhibitions. Sharing your work in progress at a time of your choosing and with a few carefully selected, supportive individuals gives you a chance to rehearse showing or performing to a larger

audience of strangers. Testing audience reaction can bolster your confidence and motivate you to complete the work. If you're getting positive feedback in the early stages, you'll be well armed by the time you show your work in public.

2. Track your work. Have a table or log for each part of your project, including at least the status and next steps for each part and also include an exhibition or performance plan. Being organized saves time and forestalls the self-sabotage that can push you away from your creative work and keep you from finishing.

3. How much do you care? Choosing projects that are deeply meaningful to you gives you the juice to stay with them until they're completed. Is there a personal milestone you'd like to achieve? Is your project going to break new ground? Which other features of your project could generate the sustained passion you'll need to complete it?

Three Tips for Coaches

1. Help your clients identify the real fear(s) that make completion a dreaded event, then help them find joy in getting to the finish line. What attitude shifts might allow them to look at completion and showing in a joyous light?

2. Investigate categorical statements (the audience won't understand, I can't talk to them, etc.). Encourage your clients to replace the negative self-talk with more motivating statements that will make them eager to complete and share their work. Ask them whether periodically showing to a friendly few could dispel some of their fears.

3. Suggest that your clients set daily and weekly intentions and adopt a new attitude of "What can I accomplish today?" Setting smaller goals more often makes things feel more doable and more enjoyable. This can help your clients develop the self-confidence and satisfaction that comes from completion.

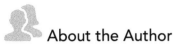 About the Author

Clare Thorbes is a certified creativity coach (clarethorbescreativitycoach.com) who works with writers, visual artists and performers. She is also a visual artist (clarethorbesfineart.com) and certified French translator. She has been published in two previous anthologies edited by Eric Maisel: *Inside Creativity Coaching* and *The Creativity Workbook for Coaches and Creatives*.

Spotlight Your Intentions

6

Cari Griffo

Intention is the artistic vision resulting from inspiration or, rather, a creative's muse. It is the beautiful flutter that activates motivation and the desire to realize an idea into fruition. Intentions for a piece of work are both large and small; they design the framework for a finished project as well as guiding the details within the process. In order to reach completion, awareness of your intentions constantly flows through your creative goals.

It is unavoidable to be thrown off track while trying to accomplish your creative work or, worse, to completely experience a drought. The fuel can disappear 100 feet underground where it once pooled to the surface. As a writer, I know this feeling and I also know for every dry spell, there are reasons for our stopping. When your energy becomes buried along the way, you lose the essence of why you started in the first place. Exploring your original vision and measuring it to where you are at now are crucial when you are stuck.

When I was writing my second novel, after making several mistakes with my first, I cautiously decided I would write the first 50 pages, then send them off to an editor for a first-read critique. Little did I know the block in flow I was setting myself up for! Instead of this new editor fulfilling my request for general notes on story development, she line edited all 50 pages. When she returned the hard copy to me, the black type was covered in bright red scribbles, smearing all 50 pages.

As a creative, you can understand how I was completely discouraged and could no longer connect to my original muse. Even though she somehow went over and beyond my request, I had to live with the consequences of my reaching out to an editor in mid-process; it was simply too soon to be consumed with an editor's details based on a first draft. A writing peer could

DOI: 10.4324/9781003351344-6

have adequately informed me about my story concept. It is important to be mindful of your actions during a creative process as there are consequences that could impede your original intention to complete the work.

Go Back

I think of the time I had a near-death experience. As I was in the tunnel of light, completely surrendering to its peacefulness, a strong voice blocked me from going any farther. "Go back," it said. "It's not time yet." Without a choice, I was pushed out of the light and as I hovered above my dead self, I was forced to trust reentering my body. Perhaps you think it's easier to allow your creative work to die, but I can tell you from experience, creations are divine and their purposes can only be discovered while alive. Before you allow your project to die, think of your stopping points as near deaths that need resuscitating.

Go back to where the idea for your work felt most alive. You must go as far backward as you can until you feel gratitude for being sent back to do your present work. A singer/songwriter client of mine came to me wanting to deepen the lyrics to a breakup song. After working too long on the lyrics, her emotional attachments became diluted; hence, the lyrics too became benign. I guided her in a visualization, taking her back to the emotions of the breakup, the muse for the song, until her entire body could feel again, until she found an ease in writing her lyrics.

Visualization is a powerful tool I use with clients to capture their original intentions. This is a condensed description:

- Get comfortable, preferably in the space you create in and close your eyes.
- Imagine yourself at the present time with your present struggle and, in your mind, cover your project with a sheet.
- Visualize walking away from your covered project, still facing it; as you continue to walk away, notice it becoming smaller.
- Remember when you first felt its conception: where you were, outside or inside; who you were with; what spurred it; how you felt; what it looked and sounded like; and so on.
- Feel your first encounter with this idea fully. Feel it now 100 times more.
- In your mind, quickly jot down your intention for this project. Feel your intention fully. Feel it now 100 times more.

Tell Your Story

One effective tool I use with clients when they are struggling to finish is role-playing: I pretend I'm a friend and ask them to tell me if they have any ideas for a new project. Phrased this way, they have an opportunity to talk about what they are working on as if they haven't started it yet. You can seek out a friend, clue them in and tell them what your intentions are for your new project. Sometimes, hearing ourselves speak the story of our work reminds us of how we got off track.

A writer I coached was stuck on page 25 of his nonfiction book but said he could visualize the entire book. While acting as his friend, I coaxed him about his project as if it wasn't in existence yet and immediately his energy lifted. Every detail of the book arose from this exercise, right down to him telling his "friend" that the entire book would be 205 pages. To emphasize what his finished book would look like, I took a 205-page book off my shelf and placed a paper clip on page 25. Then I suggested he do the same with a book at home but to design a cover for his finished book and place it on the book as a model. Once he had finally begun to write again, I suggested he move the paper clip in the book mock-up to the current page and continue doing that until he had completed the book.

Telling your story through an artistic statement is often better if you are a visual artist. Many artists only write a statement at the completion for a body of work, often upon request or for a show. To gain clarity about a roadblock, you can picture your project as if it were complete. Then you can write what you are trying to convey to your viewers, why you made certain choices along the way, or how the work has meaning for you.

What you tell them can move your work forward by defining it with words. For musicians and performers, an imaginary interview works well. Write down questions about the origin of your project, prodding questions about the muse and your motivation, or how you intend the audience to receive your work. Then answer them as if you were live on TV with thousands of viewers you are trying to impress. To deepen the experience, you can have someone else ask you the questions in a mock interview. While under the spotlight, your answers can heat up the completion of your work.

Dig Up Your Personal Attachments

Our personal attachments can be what defines our work, what makes us unique and what motivates our creativity. Like most relationships, our attachments can eventually be taken for granted and can lie quietly, waiting for us to notice them again. It is easy for creators to forget what drove them in the first place, only to lose their momentum at some point.

One of my coaching clients was obsessed with spirals. She drew them, painted them and sewed them and they turned up in every single image she made for years. When the pandemic struck and she had more time than ever available for her art, for some reason, she stopped her spirals and therefore her art, altogether. She came to me because there was a hole in her life, something she was deeply missing and furthermore, she sensed her work with spirals wasn't finished yet. She found herself starving for her own self-expression.

There are three key components to recognizing your attachments to your work. First, I worked with her on *acknowledging* what the spirals meant to her and she discovered that they were a means for healing trauma. The irony was that she had worked very hard on her healing and felt she had shifted to a healthy place. She was then able to recognize the spirals as her spirituality and could sense how her spirituality was missing in her life. *Acknowledge* what your work means to you and your intentions will flow back into your project.

The second part is *acceptance*, accompanied by giving away your work in order for others to receive it. In the spiral client's situation, she made greeting cards with bright, colorful spirals and gave them to friends. This reciprocity leads to *gratitude*: you feel fulfilled and your audience feels grateful. My spiral client completed a project I helped her set out to do with gorgeous spiral screen-printed flags, which she intended to retail. Her soul began to fly again when completing her spiral project. Your personal attachments can be the positive traits you bring to your work; *acknowledgement, acceptance* and *gratitude* are the drivers behind completing your work.

 Three Tips for Creatives

1. Write out your intentions for a new project upon the first appearance of the muse. If you haven't done so, go back anytime during the process.
2. Repeat often, "What are my intentions here?"
3. Validate your own personal attachments to your work.

Three Tips for Coaches

1. Discuss any disruptions to your client's flow that can interrupt completion.
2. Evaluate what exercises are appropriate for either going backward or forward to re-energize your client's project.
3. Assist in the discovery of your client's attachments so as to help them remember what makes their creativity unique.

About the Author

Cari Griffo (www.carigriffo.com) is a published poet with two full-length poetry books to her credit. She is also a produced and award-winning screenwriter. She holds a degree in social work and is a creativity coach, assisting innovators, musicians, visual artists, writers and performers of all ages in reaching their creative goals. She also offers expanded services to creative writers. Cari lives in the old rustic mining town of Cerrillos outside Santa Fe, New Mexico. She shares her life with her fine-art painter husband and their multitalented actress/singer-songwriter/artist daughter. She and her husband own and operate Trent Gerard Edwards Studio/Gallery in the village of Cerrillos.

How an Accountability Partner Helped Me Finish My Book

7

Shannon Borg

My longtime poet friend Kevin and I met for lunch periodically, to catch up, chat about art (my world), gossip about brewers (his world), talk about books (our shared passion) and, more often than not, whine about how we weren't writing enough or finishing the poems, books, or projects we wanted to complete.

He was always talking about wanting to simply create a daily writing practice so he could start writing regularly again. And I was always talking about my half-baked book idea: *26 Kitchens*, a food memoir about every kitchen I'd ever lived in. The problem was, although I'd written some of the "kitchens," I'd let so many other things get in the way of finishing it that the number had grown to more like 36 ten years later. I'd moved a lot, traveled a lot.

"This is embarrassing," I said over lunch, running through the kitchens in my mind, adding up the chapters, the years. "But this book won't leave me alone."

This particular day, I'm not sure what overtook me, but as I pulled away in my car, I stomped on the brakes and hung out the window to call to him on the corner, "Let's start a writing group – just you and me!"

"Sure, sure!" he laughed as he waved me off.

His unenthusiastic response might have been what spurred me on, but I called and set up a time. It was so odd. We were already writers, both writing, but the idea of a "group" somehow made us both take ourselves more seriously. I wanted to see his best work. And I wanted to see mine.

And so it began.

DOI: 10.4324/9781003351344-7

We started meeting in person, every Tuesday night at my apartment, with soda and cheese (no wine or beer – I'd been in writing groups like that before, where each session became a sloshy party).

We each brought whatever we had written that week.

No big deal, no new news. Writing groups happen all over the world, 24-7. We proceeded apace.

But as the weeks passed, as COVID hit and our meetings moved to the phone, every Sunday morning at 10:00 a.m., we both realized that this group was more than the sum of its parts.

It was the container – the boat – that would float us down this river.

And it was not just about writing but about recovery from *not* writing. About coaching each other and holding each other accountable for our commitments. About responding with honesty and support.

He worked on his daily process, poem by poem. I worked on my book, chapter by chapter.

We joked about naming our mini-group of two. We threw around logo ideas and taglines for fun. Good ways to avoid our work, good ways to start up the brain engine.

And eight months in, we finally named ourselves: the Co-Dependables. We both knew we were in recovery from our codependent relationship with writing, with our own egos, with our self-concepts of ourselves as writers. So it fit. And it stuck.

And week by week, month by month, we wrote.

At first, I brought the few chapters I'd already written from *26 Kitchens*. My childhood home. My first college dorm. My first apartment. Fun, but I knew I wasn't pushing myself and Kevin's attention helped me realize: I wanted to write the truth – my way.

And so I started, timidly at first, to write about the hard stuff: family drama, divorce, drinking. All the things that I had been afraid to write about. Kevin made me feel that it was okay to venture there.

I set them up. I knocked them down. Sometimes, knowing I had to read (out loud) to Kevin – over the phone, mind you – I would set my timer at 9:00 a.m. and rattle out two twenty-five minute sessions (or "Pomos" as we call them – from the Pomodoro Technique by Francesco Cirillo, who started this method by setting a tomato-shaped timer; I bought one for each of us).

Then I'd read what I wrote and, after group, spend three hours editing it into something real.

I created sticky notes with the list of my chapter names on them and a little box that I could check off. Such a feeling of satisfaction! Those sticky notes became my drug. The black Sharpie, the check mark, the line through the task. Bliss.

You know what I mean.

I finished the first read through – all 26 chapters. Then I started over and read the new version with my edits and his suggestions.

How to Make a Group Work for You

So, as you embark on this adventure with the goal of completing your project, I suggest these five steps:

The Steps

1. Take the leap. Start now. Don't wait. Find one other person who needs accountability, across the street or across the globe and start.
2. Get committed. Set a time and show up, no matter what. Even if you don't have anything. Even if you just want to whine. Something will come of just showing up. And beyond that, make your Post-it notes and to-do lists, even if you have made them 1,000 times before and failed to finish. You can do it and you will.
3. Tell the truth your way. The main thing that gets in the way of finishing – or even writing – is the internal fear that our very personal story – our self – is not interesting, not worthy, not worth creating. But when you can commit to telling your story your way, you know it will be unique and the freedom and self-confidence to tell it will emerge.
4. Rinse and repeat. Stick to the schedule as lives and schedules change. Think about the next idea and the next. When you get the idea for the next book, do a couple of Pomos on it and squirrel it away so you have something new to start on. Hemingway did this when he ended each day's writing session midsentence, so he had something to work on when he clocked in again.
5. Take time to celebrate. Kevin and I will be doing a book-release party in spring 2023 in Seattle at the brewery he works at. We will launch his poetry website and I will sign copies of my book. And we will marvel at the four years of Sundays we've spent in the Co-Dependables, writing, sharing, laughing and coaching each other toward our goals. It has been 100% worth every minute.

A Note on Reading Aloud

In my first class as a new poetry MFA student at the University of Washington, my professor (and venerable poet) David Wagoner started the class by reading – out loud, for three hours – ALL of Mother Goose. Or so it seemed.

He read nursery rhymes to us for three hours.

And by the end – and every week after – as he read more and more complex poems, with more and more complex rhythms, to the group, I could *hear* the new poems in my head, resonating against the scrim of sound of the nursery rhymes. After that, I read *everything* aloud, many times, as I wrote, hearing the music and the magic, looking for sour notes and wrong words.

So my dear friend Kevin listened to me read 26 chapters of my (slowly improving, sometimes clunky, sometimes successful) book. Twice. Bless him.

And I listened to him.

Now I read him everything. I even read him this chapter and he had great comments; some I used and some I left.

This is what art is and does for us. It is music that touches parts of our brains and hearts that nothing else can. And when we spend the time listening to each other as we crawl over the boulders and get our horns stuck in the hedgerows, it becomes art.

Next spring, we will celebrate with a reading. Kevin's poetry and my book release party – at the brewery, with the beer and the friends and family. We may even cry a little bit.

Because we did it. Together.

 Three Tips for Creatives

The "Time It, Type It, Tweak It" Method for Finishing Fast

1. Time it. Set a timer and write it out, record it, or type it.
    A timer gives you an end point – this agony won't go ON AND ON! You can do ANYTHING for twenty to twenty-five minutes, right? The funny thing is, once you get writing, you often go past the timer. I have even not realized the timer went off and kept writing for an hour (only sometimes).

By setting a timer for twenty to twenty-five minutes, you can focus on the thing for a short period of time – then call it GOOD. Read through it or don't, but set it aside until the next day or at least for an hour or so. I also suggest writing this out by hand the first time, for several reasons. You get more connected to your writing in a visceral, emotional way. Just channel your inner poet and go. Now, if the writing-by-hand thing makes you gag, go ahead and type or even record-to-text yourself talking (maybe for a shorter period of time). Whatever it takes to focus on this for a few minutes and get it down.

2. Type it. The reason I'm suggesting that you start out in longhand is that by writing by hand, you have a more visceral connection to the thing, the piece of writing itself. (Of course, you can also type it or record it, whatever is easier.) And then, when you type it into the computer and become "all business" about it, you can edit as you go, fix things and tweak things. Doing the two tasks separately helps you get a little distance from it. Then put all three paragraphs together and read it through a few times. Call it good for a while. Put it up on your website, print it out, let it sit for a few hours or a few days, depending on what it is. Read it again out loud and make a tweak or two.

3. Tweak it. Make the last edits and call it good. Seriously.

Notice I'm not suggesting that you get someone else to read it or take it to a group mastermind or anything like that.

I want you to trust yourself on this one.

Remember, this is YOUR art, YOUR writing, YOUR blog post, novel, memoir, artist's statement, or whatever it is. It is a living document, always in flux. You can move on and go back if you feel the need to.

Just let it sit – let it GO.

Some Ways to Let It Sit and Let It GO:

- Print out your piece and post it on a wall. Read it through out loud.
- Put it up on a page on your website (live or not live) with a good picture of you at work in your studio or whatever. Use it! If you want to change it later, you can – it is YOURS.
- Keep your writing in a folder on your computer, preferably in the cloud, like on Dropbox, Evernote, Files, etc., so you can access

it anywhere. Take it out and look at it once a week or whenever you need to.

- Write edits on the hard copy. Then type them in. This is old school, but it helps you keep your operator hat on and not get confused.
- At the very end (don't get caught up in this earlier in the process), use Grammarly or some other digital tool to make sure there are no typos.

Move on! You have a life to live and more books to write!

 Three Tips for Coaches

1. Thoughts first, then action. Ask your clients to write down their thoughts about their project. If they are lost in thoughts such as "I'll never finish this project," or "Why is this so hard?" then their actions will reflect this and will likely be actions of avoidance and resistance. If they can shift their thoughts to something more helpful, such as "I am a writer who works a little bit every day so as to be accountable to my project and myself," then their actions will likely be more productive.
2. Identify obstacles and create strategies around them. Let your clients identify their one to three main obstacles to finishing their project. Use each of these obstacles to create a strategy. For instance, if their obstacle is "not enough time," then a strategy might be to "schedule specific times on my calendar to work on a specific chapter or part of the project."
3. Make it new with emotion since emotion drives ALL our action. Sometimes clients just "get bored" with their project and "don't want to finish it." If you ask them why they don't want to finish, it is usually because they "aren't excited" by the project anymore. Ask them to create a list of three to five thoughts that would help them become excited about their project again, such as: "When I finish this project, I will have a reading with all my friends and supporters present," or "When I finish this project, I will be proud of myself for having accomplished this goal."

About the Author

Shannon Borg is an art and business coach, writer (MFA Poetry, UW/PhD Poetry, U Houston) and painter (Gage Academy of Art). She is the author of three books: *Corset* (poems), *Chefs on the Farm* and *The Green Vine*. She lives in Friday Harbor in the San Juan Islands of Washington State.

Completion

8

Journey or Destination?

Alia Thabit

When I travel, my motto is "Whatever happens is the exact right thing." Flight delays? Exact right thing. Detained by Israeli security forces? Exact right thing. Taxi breaks down in Jordanian desert and the other passenger and I have to hitchhike to the airport? Exact right thing. It helps me stay upbeat and cheerful, despite any . . . detours. I have a clear intention to reach my destination – *while* appreciating the journey as it unfolds, however unexpectedly.

When I proposed this chapter, I suggested that Somatic Experiencing® (SE), a gentle, effective trauma resolution model, could help reduce artists' challenges in finishing work as fears, resistance and anxiety are often trauma related. I'm an SE practitioner as well as a creativity coach. To explore this, I developed a ten-week group coaching program that included SE grounding skills along with my most reliable methods for getting work done. I christened it Finishing's Cool and dropped a note in my newsletter inviting readers to join me. Four artists responded and we began our journey.

The Program

We focused on developing quality habits (via tinyhabits.com), consistent time blocks for creative work, strategies for leveraging and enhancement of willpower and daily accountability made easy with a smartphone app. It included group coaching meetings and individual SE sessions. Each meeting, we checked in, troubleshot obstacles and planned our targets for the following

DOI: 10.4324/9781003351344-8

meeting. We closed with SE grounding work to soothe everyone's nervous systems.

Pre-start, I asked everyone about the current situation of their chosen project, their obstacles and what they'd like to accomplish in our time together. Our four artists (not their real names) responded.

- Gini: Finish a dance costume, a solo dance, a group choreography, or maybe all three. She wasn't sure which. Gini's chronic illness left her with little energy. Her best time went to her paying job. By evening, she was generally exhausted. Gini cited a history of starting classes and projects and then abandoning them.
- Atara: Finish her herbal certification homework. She had done all the reading. She used the material daily, but the written responses had been hanging over her for the past nine years. A single parent during summer vacation managing an herbal business and gardens to supply it, Atara was spinning a LOT of plates; time and focus were a challenge.
- Cara: Finish sewing a pair of harem pants. Cara's demanding job and PhD program left little time or energy to spare for creative work, plus she had no suitable workspace, she was a beginning seamstress and her machine didn't work properly.
- Galene: Finish a book proposal for her memoir. With a solid plan for her proposal, pieces of it already under her belt, a deadline and an agent waiting, Galene was considerably further along than the other participants. But, like them, she had been struggling . . .

I asked each artist, "What is the ONE thing you can do this week, such that by doing it, everything else will become easier or unnecessary?" (*The One Thing*, Gary Keller and Jay Papasan).

Atara decided to do laundry and clean the house so she could concentrate without distractions. Cara took her sewing machine in for repairs. Galene, already part of a daily Zoom writing group, asked her group mates to add a half hour to the period, so she had a full ninety minute block of time to write. Gini chose to gather all her costume materials and find a place to lay them all out. Then we developed habit chains for each artist, with anchor activities and designated times, places and processes to get from there to the creative work session, with a focus on celebrating each step.

We sailed into our first meeting. As with so many creative projects, we started out with plenty of motivation and early success. Everyone was completing their prep work, plus testing and refining their Tiny Habits anchors and behavior.

The Obstacles

Cara needed a different bobbin (and then a special hemmer). Galene's first chapter summary was dauntingly, hugely complex. She took a few days to breathe. Gini lacked space and energy. Atara's house never seemed to get clean. Nor was I immune – health stuff distracted me and some nudging fell by the wayside.

Yet Somehow, Things Happened . . .

- Galene returned to her project with new fire, *completing* piece after piece.
- Gini and her partner attacked their basement with hammers and sheet-rock, carving out a beautiful workspace, *complete* with plenty of storage for creative projects and a big, beautiful table to work on them.
- Atara sat down and *completed* the writing for one entire herbalism lesson – in one sitting.
- Cara used her habit skills and the new morning space she'd created to work on a scientific article she had begun with her college lab mates three years previously. Over the next few weeks, they *completed* the article and submitted it for publication – the day before one lab mate gave birth!

The upshot?

Structure for the Win!

Success came from the structure: of habits, willpower, accountability, grounding, group meetings and permission to focus on one task. Every participant cited these elements. But it also came from holding that clear intention: the destination. Completing the work.

For Gini, the frustration of NOT having a space for her projects pushed her to create one. As soon as her space was finished, she completed the group dance for an upcoming company recital. Accountability was key, especially the celebration piece and the habit work. She said, "It is so much easier to succeed when the bar is so low."

Atara faced enormous challenges as a low-income single parent. Yet when she defied the call of the house, set a work time and stuck to it, she succeeded.

Though disappointed at completing only one lesson, this small success was proof that she could do it.

Cara was thrilled to finish her scientific article. Going forward, she gave that morning space she had created to her PhD course reading, which had been proving difficult. She said, "To focus on one thing at a time and quiet the other thoughts by writing them down [and] to take my sewing one small stitch at a time resonated with me. I have easily applied this to other areas."

Galene's existing structure and determination gave her the framework to keep going. By the end of our project, she handed a full draft to her agent. She found the SE grounding skills and permission to focus on just this one task to be helpful in powering through the work at hand.

Participants found the regular group meetings and daily accountability especially helpful. Atara felt the group and consistent support helped her find determination. Gini said, "That I was accountable to you was different from all the other things that I signed up for and didn't do. I knew we had the check-ins, I knew you were sending me emails that you wanted me to respond to, you had the habit-share app – I couldn't just do nothing."

The Exact Right Thing?

Despite unexpected detours, everyone completed something important to them – from an entire project to a full chunk of a larger project. As Gini pointed out, sometimes "you have to do side quests to complete the main quest." And the intention of *completion* drove each choice.

I learned a lot. I had front-loaded the group with multiple strategies – too many to digest at once. In the future, I will piece them out so each meeting has a new tool and each tool gets to be appreciated, practiced and integrated. I would also do weekly meetings to keep group spirits high and facilitate connection between participants. Even so, what a success!

Everyone gained skills they can now bring to any project in the future – including Somatic Experiencing® grounding skills. We practiced these in every group meeting; multiple participants cited them as helpful in their ability to face their work. Though few opted for personal sessions during the project, several expressed interest in future sessions, a promising outcome for my initial theory. The seeds are planted and the sprouting has begun!

The exact right thing.

Three Tips for Creatives

1. Make daily space for the muse. Tinyhabits.com is your friend. Create a process of accountability – to a friend, a coach, your adoring fans; people who post regular progress reports are 79% more likely to succeed. Remember to celebrate each and every win, even the tiniest!
2. Decide in advance what you will work on each day (ideally, the night before). Devote your best time block to your creative work. More is great, but the first one, when you're freshest, is ideal. Ninety minutes is about max. Take breaks between blocks. Persevere: the finish line is in sight!
3. Give yourself permission to focus on this task only. All the other things will immediately start shrieking for attention. Write them down on a piece of paper as they pop up so you don't have to remember them. Tell them they are on the list and they can relax now. See AliaThabit.com/permission for a downloadable certificate you can print out and place in your workspace.

Three Tips for Coaches

1. Meet regularly. Frequency and consistency help sustain that intention of completion, as does the group ethos, for everyone supports and appreciates each other's journeys.
2. Facilitate daily scheduled work sessions. A consistent time block goes a long way toward consistent work. Scheduled daily practice made all the difference to our participants.
3. Accountability is key. Do nudge (not nag) and check in between meetings. Ask for updates, ask for obstacles and help your artists find their preferred way around these obstacles. If they can't, then suggest something for them to play with.

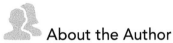 ## About the Author

Alia Thabit is an Arab American creativity coach, belly dancer, artist, author and Somatic Experiencing® (SE) practitioner. She champions self-expression, resilience and trust in the body. Alia is the author of *Midnight at the Crossroads: Has Belly Dance Sold Its Soul?* a book about the surprising depths of the dance. Her work helps clients reclaim their joyful spirit and deep wells of creativity so they can bring joy to the world. An international and online presenter with decades of experience, Alia is available for coaching and more at AliaThabit.com.

Three Steps to Perseverance

9

Nick Lazaris

Persistence is defined as the quality that allows someone to continue doing something even though it is difficult or frustrating when obstacles, whether external or internal, appear. It is probable that your lack of perseverance is connected to negative self-talk that causes doubt in what you are creating and hoping to complete.

Maybe you're not persistent because you are afraid of what others might think. Other times, things are simply difficult and it becomes hard to keep moving forward through the challenge. In fact, the more you actually go for your goals as a creative, the greater the probability that you might struggle at some point with being persistent in your journey toward completion. This is because a lack of persistence is most often fear based and to keep pushing forward can lead to anxiety and stress.

The question is, "Do you persevere when times get tough or when you are under pressure to complete your work?"

Jonathan and Perseverance

A new client, whom I'll call Jonathan, came to me while writing the final chapters of his book on music theory. Although he truly believed that there was a need for such a book for music students, Jonathan found himself "stuck" completing his book and could not understand why. He had hit a roadblock and had become discouraged as he found his everyday writing slowing down as he moved away from his commitment to complete his book.

I shared with him how football legend Vince Lombardi described the importance of perseverance when he said, "The difference between a successful

DOI: 10.4324/9781003351344-9

person and others is not a lack of strength, nor a lack of knowledge, but rather a lack of will." I was suggesting to Jonathan that his excuses and rationalizations were preventing him from completing his work and were masking the real struggle he was experiencing.

Together, we uncovered that the obstacle to completing his book was based on his fear of what others might say about his book. Jonathan realized that his self-doubt had been screaming (or sometimes quietly suggesting) that he was not good enough to become a successful writer.

Phrases such as "Who do I think I am to be writing this book?" and "Will anyone really buy it?" came to the surface as we gently stripped away the subconscious excuses that were the basis for his lack of perseverance.

Through understanding the following three steps to creating a mindset that supported perseverance, Jonathan was able to say, "Yes, I have all of the strength, talent and ideas I need to keep moving forward. Now it's time to remove my negative mindset and finish the book."

Perseverance became a key part of his commitment to his writing goals, not on a one-time basis, but rather daily, hourly and continually.

These powerful steps lead to greater focus, stronger motivation, reduced stagnation and, most importantly, increased perseverance.

Step #1 – Stop Talking and Start Doing!

Mark Twain once said, "Noise [talking] proves nothing. Often a hen who has merely laid an egg cackles as if she had laid an asteroid."

Perseverance in your creative life is not achieved through hoping, wishing, or just talking about it but through persistent effort, action and consistent commitment to your passion and goals on a continuous basis.

How often do we wish for what we want, or talk about it, rather than going out and getting it? It is vital to make an intentional choice to commit yourself to that which you desire through action and perseverance. Remember that talk is cheap and action is king!

Step #2 – Never Wait for the "Perfect Time"

Those who are mentally tough as creators *create* opportunity. They take responsibility for their creative life and career.

Yes, taking risks leads to taking charge of one's work. Assert yourself when necessary and stop blaming anything inside or outside you if your creative project doesn't go the way you desire in the time you want. Many people who desire success always seem to be "getting ready" to do the work, rather than actually doing the task that is right in front of them. In fact, sometimes you might even find yourself getting ready to get ready!

Are you letting fear or the desire to "get it just right" keep you from starting? Think about what you would accomplish if you practiced persistence, stopped aiming for perfection and instead committed to doing *something* consistently, even if it isn't perfect or exactly the way you believe it should be.

Begin to quiet that fearful inner voice you hear saying, "Well, I tried, but it didn't work out. I guess I'll stop and pursue something else." Persistence involves giving your goals enough time to actually be achieved. "If you wait for perfect conditions, you will never get anything done" (Ecclesiastes 11:4).

Step #3 – Overcome Your Fear of Rejection and Failure

The main reason creatives do not stay persistent and give up too soon is the fear that they may fail or be rejected.

Of course, no one likes rejection. Yet, as we know, *yes* lives in the land of *no*. The more *nos*, or obstacles, you experience, the more likely it is that you are asking for what you want, trying new ideas and stretching yourself through risking new ways of creating.

The "What ifs?" in our thinking, which lead to our looking ahead in anxious anticipation, will also ruin any chance of experiencing the present moment, especially during times of taking the risk of working toward completion with persistence.

Until you are willing to say, "So what? My creative dreams matter to me!" and keep pursuing the thing that you desire until completion, your lack of perseverance will derail you.

So often we miss what is right in front of us by nervously looking ahead in fear. Learning to say, "So what?" as you step out of fear and take the next action step will take you closer to achieving your goal.

Do you give up too soon? Henry Wadsworth Longfellow said, "Perseverance is a great element of success. If you only knock long enough and loud enough at the gate, you are sure to wake up somebody."

A commitment to focusing on and working toward achieving the goals that truly matter to you is not a straight line – there will be ups and downs, successes and limitations, throughout your creative journey.

The world needs you to hang in there, to not give up, to persevere with your amazing book, piece of art, or potential world-changing idea.

I encourage you TODAY to make a choice to commit yourself to completing your work through action, hard work and, most importantly, perseverance

 Three Tips for Creatives

1. Stop talking and start doing! The moment you realize that you are not persevering in your work, immediately commit yourself to a very specific action step. It doesn't matter what it is – do something connected to the work while telling yourself, "It's time to take some action." Remind yourself that wishing, hoping and talking are cheap. Only taking action matters

2. Never wait for the "perfect time." Challenge the inner voice that desires to get your project just right but keeps you from actually completing the work. Remind yourself, "The only thing that matters is to do the next step that is right in front of me."

3. Overcome your fear of rejection and failure. "What if it's not perfect?" must be replaced with "So What?" thinking – "I can do this and I'm going to complete my work and move forward from here."

 Three Tips for Coaches

1. Encourage your client's self-awareness by helping "peel back the layers" of critical, internal messages. Gently but firmly point out the rationalizations and excuses that cover up their true fears of failure and rejection.

2. Remind your client that the reality of a "perfect time" does not exist – it is simply the mind's powerful way of putting off potential rejection, a sort of kicking the can of failure down the road.

3. Help your client develop a heightened awareness of and listen for any thinking that includes "What if?" and create an immediate follow-up of "So what? I am going to do the next thing right in front of me."

About the Author

As a performance psychologist and creativity coach, Dr. Nick Lazaris has specialized for 38 years in helping creatives, performing artists, entrepreneurs and business professionals overcome anxiety in their art, writing, or public speaking or while onstage. Dr. Nick coaches those who desire to increase their self-confidence, overcome fear and create at or near their personal best. Contact him at nick@drnicklazaris.com or go to www.drnicklazaris.com to receive your free Performance Anxiety Road Map.

A Mindful Approach to Completing Creative Work

10

Thomas Deneuville

Coaches are all too familiar with the reasons creatives don't complete their work. From not knowing when to stop to shiny-object syndrome or spending too much time researching a project, there seems to be an endless list of traps creatives fall into while attempting to finish their most meaningful projects.

While, arguably, some reasons fall under logistics or timing and consequently feel out of the creative's control, the common denominator in many traps is the creative's own mind. Their relationship with their mind, to be precise, is a critical element at every stage of the creative process, especially near completion.

The double bar, the final brushstroke, or the last word can seem to come at a great price. As a creative nears completion, their fears can launch a final offensive and flood their mind with a deluge of excuses – some even deceptively rational – to prevent them from completing their work. Amid these anxieties, it takes a trained mind to focus on the work, a mind imbued with fearlessness or creative warriorship. This training starts with simple steps, the most important one being practicing mindfulness meditation.

Mindfulness can be defined as paying attention to the present moment and noticing what arises without bias or judgment. In other words, learning to stay with what is – whether it's pleasant or not. Curious, transformative things happen when we stay with what is. As an example, let me tell you about Melanie.

Melanie was a historical fiction writer who came to me for coaching because she couldn't complete her novel. During our introductory call, she told me that she had already tried to write two novels but had abandoned

DOI: 10.4324/9781003351344-10

them: with her first book, she fell out of love with the protagonists, while with her second, she discovered that the idea had already been written and published by another author.

After a couple of sessions, Melanie had established a new writing schedule that fit better with her day job and had defined micro goals to build momentum on her first draft. At the end of one of our calls, out of curiosity, I asked her if she meditated. "Only during yoga classes," she replied, "but I could use some help dealing with the stress of my day job." We ended our session with a ten-minute guided meditation in which I shared a simple three-step method and I encouraged her to add meditation to her routine.

Months went by and Melanie was making good progress on her novel. Something unexpected happened, though. During her writing sessions, familiar thoughts would come and visit her: "This novel is going nowhere. . . . I'm not a writer." These were the same thoughts that had led her to abandon two novels, but this time something was different. Melanie more often felt *detached* from these thoughts. They didn't hurt like the truth or seduce her like lies; Melanie just noticed them with curiosity and went back to work.

At first, this was confusing. "Am I losing interest in writing?" she asked during our next session. But I credited this shift to her mindfulness meditation practice and invited her to keep up the good work. We soon decided that she didn't need my help anymore and Melanie completed her novel ten months later.

Melanie committed to her writing and put a lot of time and effort into completing her novel. She also experienced firsthand the benefits of mindfulness meditation. Contrary to popular belief, her sitting practice didn't put her in a state of peaceful bliss. She still struggled with the same thoughts that had defeated her in the past, but she was learning to stay present with them without judgment or attachment. Like clouds in the sky, these thoughts passed and she could keep on writing.

But mindfulness has other appealing qualities for creatives besides bringing them back to their work when distracted by discursive thoughts. Indeed, mindfulness is a gateway to a path of fearless creativity or creative warriorship.

Warriorship here must not be construed as aggression, though. In the Shambhala teachings, warriorship refers to a tradition of individual bravery found across cultures and eras (for example, Amazons and Samurai). Creative warriorship, then, is a series of realizations and practices (including mindfulness meditation) that lead creative individuals to form a deep, intimate knowledge of their fears – the proverbial "the only way out is through."

Thankfully, studies have shown that newcomers see the benefits of mindfulness meditation (clarity, stability, strength, etc.) within months, if not weeks. It is never too early – or too late – for a creative to consider mindfulness-based contemplative practices and I would like to offer three tips for creatives, as well as three tips for coaches.

Three Tips for Creatives

1. When trying to reconnect with your work to complete it, it can be helpful to anchor yourself in your body. Traditionally, in mindfulness meditation, the vehicle is the breath. When you focus on it, you synchronize your body and your mind and achieve a grounding sense of stillness and presence. If you experience some emotional distress, focusing on the breath might not be enough and you might want to try the five-four-three-two-one technique. After taking a few deep breaths, unhurriedly notice five things you can see, followed by four things you can touch, three things you can hear, two things you can smell and, finally, one thing you can taste. Take a few deep breaths and return to your work.

2. Often, what stands between you and the work is a tangle of discursive thoughts and it is worth trying to provide a mindful outlet for them. Before starting to work on your creative project, take a few pieces of scrap paper. At the top of the first one, write: "Why can't I complete [fill in the name of creative project]?" Write down the first reason that comes to mind. Don't judge it, don't comment on it; just write it down. Try to be as curious as possible and every time you feel like you've reached a new block, ask yourself, "Yes, but why?" Be an observer and try not to hold on to or reject any reasons that you write down. When you feel like you've exhausted the reasons you can't complete your work, crumple up the pages, throw them in the closest recycling bin and return to your work.

3. My third tip is to embrace work as meditation. Focus your attention on the sensations of your medium to reduce the pull of distracting thoughts: the clicking of your keyboard's keys, the resistance of the rosined bow's hair against the strings, the clay spinning between your fingers. This will feel a bit strange because in mastering your skill, you probably started paying *less* attention to some details.

You might even make some novice mistakes. But soon, you'll find a reliable anchor for your attention and whenever you find your mind racing ahead or getting caught in discursive thoughts ("This is bad," or "I should start from scratch"), bring your attention back to your medium to complete your work. Be gentle, though. You are not blaming yourself for having such thoughts. You're simply noticing them – you could even label them "thinking" – and then bringing your attention back to your medium, where the work happens.

 Three Tips for Coaches

1. Model for your client what a mindful approach to life looks like. Start your sessions with a mindful minute or a few deep breaths. Invite your client to take a brief pause when they've just shared a powerful thought with you or when a pause begs to linger. Helping clients focus more on the process than on the outcome is also a fundamentally mindful strategy: everything (including creation) can only happen in the *now*.

2. Help your clients establish a meditation practice. If you are trained as a meditation teacher, consider offering instructions during your sessions. If you aren't, invite your client to take classes or retreats. Make it clear that meditation shouldn't be pursued to become a better creative but to see themselves and their creative practice as they are and to become friends with themselves.

3. As coaches, we acknowledge the challenges that our clients face when struggling to complete their creative work and we validate their feelings. But we also help them expand their perspectives. My preferred way is through humor. When appropriate – and always with kindness – offering to laugh about a situation can surprise a client. Like a Zen paradox, humor can challenge the way they think and lead to some unexpected creative solutions or at least to a softening or an opening of some sort.

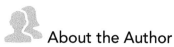 ## About the Author

Thomas Deneuville is a creativity coach and mindfulness meditation teacher. He draws on 15 years of meditation practice and his classical training in voice and composition to help his clients achieve their creative goals and take their first steps on the path of creative warriorship. He lives in Freeville, NY, with his wife, two sons and a growing collection of bagpipes.

Planting Your Work   11

Midori Evans

Growing a garden is a labor of love made up of pruning, tending, deadheading, soil amendments and more. Even with our best intentions, the unknowns associated with caring for a garden are many: scourges of beetles, an early season windstorm that takes out the peonies, the dreaded gray mold. We may never get our garden looking quite as good as we may wish. Yet we gardeners all persevere, buying that one special fertilizer or reshaping the topiary for the hundredth time.

What does all this have to do with finishing a creative project? Isn't this book about getting to that point where it really IS done, where we can dispense with our play, our choreographed dance, our final book chapter? People's creative projects grow much the same way that plants do. As they take in the amazing warmth and energy of the sun, our projects emerge, bubble up and fill us with inspiration. But it's the doubts that kill them, as if we needed to manufacture pests, drought, or the drooping leaves of a hot summer day. We get stuck finishing our work, stopping the growth process through the force of our will or merely a lack of attention.

The parallels between creative completion and caring for a garden lie in how we frame our thinking. Just as we aggressively treat a rampaging fungal infection amongst the tomatoes, we must examine what thought patterns are preventing us from considering our work done. Plants are never "fully done," and neither are our creative projects. But we can complete those projects and joyfully release them to the universe, much as we appreciate the beauty of the gardens around us.

Have you ever had the experience of bewailing a lack of progress on a project, only to finally look at it and realize that much more was done than you had imagined? Or do you lie awake nights wondering how you can reach a required word count but then find it easier to do once you finally get down to work?

DOI: 10.4324/9781003351344-11

Consider what is keeping you from finishing your work.

1. Do you think there would be a better word, color, or dance move if only you could make it happen?
2. Do you fear judgment of your finished work so you believe it better not to complete it?
3. Are there working steps, such as clearing your to-do list, that would allow you to move on?

Now envision your work within a "growing your garden" framework. Pair these questions with the following:

1. Have you ever looked at a flower and thought, "Why isn't it a different color?"
2. When you are planning a new place for a plant or experimenting with a new choice, do you ever think, "I should not look at this garden because it is not done?"
3. Think of a time when you have truly appreciated the beauty of a blooming flower or the lovely greenery of a healthy tree. In that moment, was the flower bloom not completely done? Did you find yourself thinking, "If only this bloom were slightly to the left or more purple?" Of course not! You loved and appreciated it for its beauty in the moment.

How can we cultivate this type of thinking – the type of thinking that appreciates the ebb and flow of garden life? Gardeners are a lot like creative people. Compliment them on their garden and they may very well say, "Just wait until the dahlias are blooming in August!" It is as if neither they nor we creatives can appreciate the beauty of now. But gardens continue to grow and are loved, year to year. Imagine tending the garden of your creativity in the same way. You prune your project down so it can be done in its intended year, before the winter comes. Or you plan for a biennial project, knowing you need the longer two-year cycle before your ideas can fully come to fruition.

Completing a project means that we need to stop perfecting the project, move on to details necessary for submitting a project to the external world, mark the ritual between working and ending and actually let go and feel completion!

Using specific plant references can help. Think of the project you are working on right now and ask yourself how long it will be before it could be completed. Do you find yourself getting discouraged at that length of time it and using that thought to delay the work? Think of the wasabi plant. Wasabi is extremely hard to grow, is likely to get diseases when planted on a large scale and takes more than a year to reach maturity. Yet we cultivate it and Japanese cuisine depends on it.

Do you worry that you don't have the details quite right and therefore cannot finish? Are you trying to please every audience that might interact with your work? Think of the American holly plant. This plant grows slowly but presents a beautiful contrast: spiny green leaves and gorgeous red berries. The green and the red complement each other; while humans can enjoy viewing the plant, the berries are poisonous for human consumption, but birds and other mammals can eat them. So different audiences are happy with different parts of the plant!

Now ask yourself, "What will this project be like when I give it to the world? How will it be perceived?" If you can only imagine a small audience or a short period of time for your book run or a single night of a choreographed dance, picture the Queen of the Night plant, which blooms only at night with beautiful white flowers that last for a few short hours. These plants are prized for their unique beauty. The world will welcome your project!

Finally, it is time to release the work! Picture the bird of paradise plant, with its bold colors, its unusual shape and its sporadic blooms. Imagine your work standing proudly at the end of the stalk, sticking out to the world and showing off in all of its glorious colors!

 Three Tips for Creatives

1. Choose a part of the natural world that you most resonate with. If it isn't a part of a garden you are familiar with, it could be a botanical garden, the ocean, or the sky. Whatever it is, pay attention to its seasonal patterns and its fluid and cyclical nature. Write your observations in a nature journal and then pair your creative work with these shifts.
2. You are unique, just like every garden is unique. There is no garden on the planet that has the perfect arrangement: amount of sunlight, soil type, or placement. Yet the garden is there, in its individual glory, complete in the moment. Be your own garden and remember that people will be glad your creative output exists.
3. Don't be afraid to create and complete away from strict calendar time. Be with earth time, just as your garden is. Work with a completing

morning ritual matched to sunrise times instead of a regular time on the clock, or simply remind yourself that gardens shift from growth to death to renewal in an ongoing cycle. Imagine your work in the same way and know that each completed work is like a flower blooming: all the energy of the plant has gone into making a beautiful flower and then the pattern shifts, pouring energy into seed production for the next season.

Three Tips for Coaches

1. What does this feel like in real time, for a real person? Annabelle wants to run workshops but feels intimidated. She overprepares, planting far too many seeds of ideas, scattering them around disciplines and audiences, resulting in overwhelm. She lacks the framework she needs, tries to do too much and gives up. Using a gardening framework, guide her to imagine her workshops as contained within a 1,000-square-foot plot. Divide the plot into five separate 200-square-foot sections. Have her sketch out a drawing of the garden, roughly to scale and choose plots to "plant," naming each plot by workshop title or focus.

2. Next, guide her to the idea of growing grapes. Grapes take a long time to grow into fruit-producing vines. Thinking that a workshop business will just "spring up" overnight has meant that the level of discouragement is defeating the long-term goal. Have Annabelle draw out a trellis as a structure for the grape vine and label various parts: the small vine, not yet able to reach the first leg of the trellis; the fledgling vine, stretching out across the trellis but not yet producing; and so on. While doing this, play with the gardening metaphor so it is more than a list of tasks for building the business. Envision the long view of the process and work with some deep questions around how to manage the emotions when the grapes do not produce as rapidly as she might wish.

3. Keep the grape analogy over the course of the few years it takes to grow and develop the business. Once grapes are being produced, you can categorize them, just as you would categorize workshops,

retreats and other events. What are the categories? Which ones will you plant first and which will you fertilize? When grapes are ripening at the store, you can make this a full sensory experience by purchasing multiple kinds of grapes and pairing feelings, taste, promise and ambition.

 ## About the Author

Midori Evans is the founder of Midori Creativity, which is growing a nurturing ecosystem for creatives through workshops, coaching and community projects. A lifelong creative explorer, Midori draws on the inspiration of the natural world in her work as a creativity coach, writer and landscape photographer. She recently curated *Meditations on Landscape*, a text-imagery exhibit exploring how our home landscape influences our creative process. She is currently working on a year-long creative participatory writing experience in her hometown. Look for her photographic work at Cedarlightimages.com and for seasonal Artist's Way classes at midoricreativity.com.

Use Performance to Encourage Completion

12

B. Morey Stockwell

I love music. All kinds of music. Listening to the radio, watching live concerts and even making music myself. In high school, every day before classes started, my friends and I gathered in the band room, where we chatted with each other and our fearless leader and teacher, Alyn H. Platt. I fully identified with the other band nerds.

When my kids were young, I didn't care if they played sports or joined Scouts. I wanted them to learn to play an instrument and benefit from the familial advantages of playing in an orchestra or a band. My son took up the bassoon and my daughter sampled violin, flute, piano and later voice. My husband and I gladly paid for their private lessons at a nearby music school. Through this association, I got the inkling to resume playing the bass clarinet, my longtime favorite instrument, after a twenty-year hiatus.

One thing led to another and I registered for private clarinet lessons for the first time in my life. I met Paul Surapine, the founder and executive director of the Claflin Hill Symphony Orchestra, a nonprofit organization that produced live concerts in eastern Massachusetts. Our lessons were engaging, entertaining and fun.

About halfway through my first semester, Paul said, "I think you should play in a recital." What had been an amusing preoccupation that took me away from my home-based business for thirty minutes every Wednesday afternoon suddenly became a source of angst. The thought of playing before an audience seemed outrageous. But Paul added, "It's customary for students to show what they've learned in the end-of-semester recital. It will give you something to work toward." He shared with me a piece that would be challenging but doable and a great showpiece for the recital. I began to work on learning the music.

DOI: 10.4324/9781003351344-12

My at-home practice sessions immediately shifted. I left the sheet music on the stand and the instrument assembled on the chair. I had a purpose. I was motivated. I didn't want to embarrass myself or my teacher with a mediocre show. And even though I knew I wouldn't be amazing, I started to believe that I could be okay. Week after week, I practiced for thirty to forty-five minutes, even an hour or more, at least once a day. My attention gained laser focus as the date of my upcoming recital loomed.

On May 21, 1999, I performed Eugene Bozza's *Ballad for Bass Clarinet and Piano*. It was scary, exhilarating, frustrating and fantastic. That performance changed my understanding of art and, consequently, of creativity. If art is the process and performance is the product, then makers who struggle with completing a creative art project benefit from working toward the singular moment of the show.

I began to see a similar pattern in my artist friends. I knew writers who loved the process of writing and were happy to put in the hours of composing stories, novels and essays but held back when it came time to seek publication. Publishing mimics performance in many ways as a deadline often impends in the future, but it lacks the singular focus of a specific time and place for the show. However, a perceivable shift occurs when a writer participates in a reading, such as a poetry slam or a chapter reading for a writers' group. The same is true for visual artists who participate in an art show because galleries, museums and even local libraries typically kick off the show with an open public reception. The reception is a performance. The artist mingles with patrons, friends, family and guests. Often, they'll take a few minutes to talk about their art background, training and process.

The performing arts of theatre and music have long reaped the benefits of working toward the show. Still, any artist/creative/maker working in any art form also benefits from working toward a performance. A chef, a baker, or a culinary artist might dream of opening a restaurant, bakery, or food truck, but the illusive vision lacks focus. They put off that fantasy. They wonder how they can perform. Here's an idea: they could ask a friend to host a pop-up dinner at their home or apartment with the sole purpose of performing their culinary skills for an audience. Part of the show would include the chef coming out of the kitchen and speaking to those present. They share their background, their training, motivation and love of the culinary art they do. Now there's motivation to perfect their signature dish and go public.

Those working in the industrial arts, which includes woodworking, glass-blowing, metalwork and rigid materials, can also host a reveal. Perhaps they have constructed a sculpture that could be displayed at a local playground or beach. Make it a show. Enlist the local parks and recreation department and host an unveiling. Settle on a time and place, then build an audience by writing a press release and sharing it with the local media in print or online.

A landscaper cultivates a patio patch and contacts a local garden club to host a tour. The gardener talks about a specific plant or the aesthetics of visual arrangement. An interior designer remodels a kitchen and invites a small audience to learn about the process of complementary color and design. A fiber artist working in quilt art, fashion, crochet, or knitting can also benefit from a similar performance. Perhaps they could host a quilting bee at their home studio, share it with members of a local guild and demonstrate a new technique or tool. Take photos of your art and bring your lecture to the audience with a projected slideshow. Performance gives art and art making purpose and focus.

When I coach clients, we quickly begin working toward performance after learning about their interests, goals, blocks and hindrances. This self-imposed goal of performing to share their art elevates their work sessions. They ramp up their production and view their daily output – whether it is time spent, canvas area covered, or words or notes written – as incremental steps toward that performance.

Artists/creatives/makers benefit from shifting to the perspective of the imagined audience, seeing their work, hearing their work, tasting their work, touching, feeling and experiencing their work. That shift in point of view, away from the artist to the viewpoint of an audience, helps the maker see little flaws and inconsistencies. With renewed insight, they continue their work, revise, edit and cultivate with the intention of sharing that art product with an audience.

How Does the Artist/Creative/Maker Begin?

The first step: get a calendar and look ahead 30 to 60 days, depending on the project. Choose a doable date, time and venue. Ask friends to help. Would Dave's deck serve as an excellent location to debut your new burger menu? Would your favorite coffee shop host a morning lecture on portraiture? Would the nursery downtown permit a sculptor to share their carving? The gathering does not have to be large and the venue does not have to be grand. Live performance focuses the maker's attention on finishing.

If you're wondering what venues might appreciate your performance, think about local clubs, organizations and senior centers. These groups would love to have a seamstress come in and show a capsule wardrobe and how to put pieces together. Boys' Clubs, Girls' Clubs, 4-H, Scouts, senior centers, churches and civic groups will eagerly welcome a woodworker, a chef and a watercolorist to visit a meeting and share their trade. A gardener could contact their local garden supply store. The performance must be live, but it does not have to be in person. Zoom, Facebook, or YouTube Live can be outstanding virtual platforms and in this way, you could perform for a global audience. Send out your save-the-date cards or email invitations. Then begin. Don't hesitate. Act quickly. It's showtime, folks.

When I performed my first solo recital, I did not fully realize the shift this singular focus would bring to other aspects of my life. But more importantly, the paradigm shift of transforming every art form toward a show always promotes the finishing of our creative work. Once the artist schedules the date and place, the creative announces the performance, the maker sends invitations and once the tickets are sold (even if they're free), the show must go on. After all, no one wants to show up to a sign on the door reading, "Sorry. I got distracted. I lost interest. Maybe I'll get going again next month."

 Three Tips for Creatives

1. By preparing for a performance, your efforts become sharpened and focused. Choose one creative art product that you can perform for an audience.
2. Performance elevates your art by going public, even on a small, local scale. This first step exercises your creative muscle, a necessary step regardless of your ultimate dream goal.
3. Artists/creatives/makers can perform any art form. Performances must be live, but explore virtual venues to broaden your outreach. Seek the help of friends and family. Think outside the box.

 Three Tips for Coaches

1. Ask your client what one creative art product they could perform. Brainstorm possible venues that would welcome a live presentation of the product.

2. Tackle like tasks to maximize effort. Remind the client to break out all required steps before the performance. Use a calendar to set specific dates for specific tasks.
3. Ask your client to share their "dress rehearsal" with you. Remember that your role is to support their efforts with positive feedback. Try the sandwich method. Sandwich constructive criticism between a compliment and praise for effort. Future tense your critique. Couch a suggestion with "Next time, try this."

 ## About the Author

B, Morey Stockwell teaches expository and research writing, public speaking and fashion technology at two state universities. She coaches artists/creatives/ makers and writes about creativity. Dr. Stockwell regularly posts articles on *Psychology Today*'s blog. She recently published *Do Your Art! 10 Simple Steps to Enhance Your Creativity and Elevate Your Mood*, a book on process and practice. Find more of Stockwell's valuable resources at www.doyourart.org.

How Community Can Help Solitary Creatives Finish

13

Jana Van der Veer

The popular image of the artist or writer is still one of solitary struggle in the proverbial garret, wrestling alone with the muse, in a herculean effort to create great work. It is true; to accomplish creative work we do need alone time to write, to paint, to draw, to dream.

However, artists and creatives in many disciplines benefit tremendously from being a part of an engaged community. Even if this "community" consists of just one other person who is also doing the work and who understands and supports our struggles, it encourages us to persevere through disappointments and gives us accountability to finish what we start.

I asked members of the Zoom writing group I host and the students of a course I run to support women creatives for their thoughts on a number of aspects of creative community. I asked them not just about ours but about any communities they are part of that help them in completing creative work.

From this, it emerged that challenges with finishing usually take two forms: partway through a project, when we aren't clear how to proceed and the initial enthusiasm has worn off and when we sense that the end is near, when the fear of putting our work out into the marketplace can paralyze us. (Is it good enough? How will it be received?)

Being part of a creative community can be important in overcoming our doubts and getting us to the finish line. We get mentorship, support, encouragement, contacts, knowledge, deadlines and accountability, as well as the satisfaction of being part of a group of people working seriously on their art. Our communities can help us overcome resistance, blocks and fear of failure.

DOI: 10.4324/9781003351344-13

As one writer put it,

> Almost without exception, my communities help me to complete work. One group meets weekly and I can get on a roll of presenting pages every week. Great deadlines. And they are so brilliant that they push me until the pieces are really ready. Then I present larger chunks to my monthly group. If feedback ever causes me to stumble, I have plenty of folks to help me process and find my next steps.

Of course, finding the *right* community is crucial. It must be a supportive, positive environment with good, respectful communication between members and active contributors. It should be at the right level for your work and your goals. In fact, to get the most out of any community, you must understand your goals in being part of it. Is it for professional networking? Mutual support and camaraderie? Critique? Some combination of these?

It is especially important for members of marginalized groups to find a community of peers, since they often have even more challenges in navigating creative careers. However, groups can spring up around all sorts of identities, such as race/ethnicity, gender, sexual orientation, etc. The main thing is whether or not the group understands and can support the challenges you face.

As one writer put it,

> All the wonderful women [in my] mom's writer's club were my saving grace. It was like this great Venn diagram of who I was as a person. I'd been with writer groups before, but they didn't understand that I can't just write all day. I can't. I have children. And I had groups of mom friends who didn't understand. They would say, just stop writing. Also no. That's not a thing I can do. And so, I had this great intersection in this wonderful community and it truly saved my writing and my sanity.

Although people felt overwhelmingly positive about being part of a creative community, there can be drawbacks. These include competitiveness – what one person called "compare and despair"; mean-spirited feedback; talking about the work more than doing the work; and having work derailed by a critique that is unhelpful or unskilled.

Fortunately, there are many ways to find a community that works for you. In addition to in-person options, the online world has seen an explosion of new and expanded opportunities in recent years. Even if many people prefer in-person meetings, they appreciate these ways to meet new people (including those outside their geographic area) and stay connected through pandemic, illness, motherhood, disability and other restrictions.

Some examples of creative communities include:

Accountability partner. As stated earlier, this can be just you and a friend. You can exchange actual critiques, brainstorm ideas, or just send check-in texts that say "Hey! I did my work today!" What it's good for: low-key support from someone you know has your back.

Amateur group. A group that meets around a particular discipline, such as writing or photography. This may be more for social support but often involves critiquing each other's work. What it's good for: community, support and encouragement; rarely is it best for helping you develop your craft since you may be at varying levels of experience, both in terms of the work itself and the ability to give effective critique.

Professional group. Again, this is usually organized around a particular discipline, but it is focused on professional development and opportunities to build skills, network, receive instruction and / or mentoring and so on. Examples: Society of Children's Book Writers and Illustrators, Women in Film, etc. What it's good for: networking and learning. However, you must put in the effort to get involved.

Community organization. This may be general (a local arts center) or focused on one particular creative area (a pottery collective that works out of the same facility or a community theatre, for example). What it's good for: collegial support, instruction, mentorship, collaboration and opportunities to showcase your work.

Class or workshop (in person or online). Whether ongoing or a one-off, this type of community helps you learn new skills and develop your craft. What it's good for: it may be better for beginners to intermediate practitioners. However, there is usually no ongoing support after the class ends, unless the class is part of a larger community organization.

Conference. Many different types are available, from those geared toward beginners to professional level. A web search of "your creative discipline + conference" will likely generate ideas to keep you going for years. It's important to understand what the conference is focused on: generating new work? Meeting marketplace professionals such as agents, editors, or producers? Craft instruction? What it's good for: inspiration, new knowledge of craft / industry, but often, any upswing in motivation is short lived.

MFA program. The granddaddy of serious commitments to your creative discipline. What it's good for: high-level craft development, possibility of good connections, community of high-level writers or artists. However, you may spend a lot of time critiquing others' work and the level of mentorship and teaching skill varies. It's also very expensive unless you get scholarships.

Artist/writer residency. A web search will generate numerous opportunities. Depending on the program, it may be open to many different creative disciplines or to one form only; it may be for established or emerging artists; it may support creatives from a particular region, gender, ethnicity, or some other identity. Residencies generally allow for solitude to create, as well as opportunities to share work and be part of a community. What it's good for: time away from other responsibilities to focus on creating, peer networking. Some you must pay for; others are by scholarship/fellowship application only.

Online community. Geared around a specific creative endeavor, such as sketchbookskool.com for visual artists or apex-writers.com or Manuscript Academy for writers. It may provide instruction, access to social media communities, industry and marketplace information, or other opportunities. Or it may take the form of a Zoom meetup, where everyone practices their art together (with mics and cameras on or off). These can be daily, weekly, or monthly and may be informal (everyone just hops on and does the work) or more formal, involving introductions and exchanging work.

Social media communities. Often casual but can be good sources of support, information and feedback. What it's good for: accessible community no matter where you live; other benefits depend on what's offered. You do have to actively participate to get the most out of your membership. There are, of course, plenty of social media groups that are free to join as well. The downside may be that you spend more time posting than actually working!

Creativity coach (or another professional mentor). Many creativity coaches focus on one particular area (book coach, art coach, drama coach). They offer personalized support, accountability, craft development and industry/marketplace guidance. They may help you meet a short-term goal or work with you on a long-term project (such as writing a novel). What it's good for: this will depend on the coach and their particular offerings, but generally accountability, ongoing support, project management, development of craft and knowledge of marketplace issues. However, you need to make sure you get the right person for your needs. Personality fit and coaching style and skill can mean more than stellar accomplishments in the artistic field.

Note that you don't have to have just one type of support! I have my Zoom group and a writing group of long standing; I belong to a few Facebook groups; I've taken classes and attended conferences; I've done my MFA; and I am a book coach (in a community of book coaches). You may have different needs as your career develops. As with many things, community is what you make of it. If one doesn't work for you (too toxic or not the right level), move on and know that you will eventually find your tribe.

The point is that no matter how introverted or extraverted you are, where you live, your level of experience, or how much you can afford to spend, there is some form of support, community and accountability out there for you. If you want to meet your goals and finish your creative projects, a community, no matter how small, can be your greatest ally.

 Three Tips for Creatives

1. You may need different types of community at different stages in your career. Look at the list provided here. What types of community appeal to you? Are you looking for peer support? A mentor or coach? A class to build new skills? Think about a couple you could research.
2. When you are trying to finish a big project, communities can support you or hinder you. Communities can provide accountability as well as support for finishing, but don't let your involvement in a community (or communities) distract you from actually doing the work!
3. Don't be afraid to leave a community if it doesn't feel like a good fit. Be respectful, but don't assume that others, even those further along in their careers than you, know better than you do about your work or career. On the flip side, be a positive, engaged member of any communities you commit to.

 Three Tips for Coaches

1. Encourage your clients to become part of one or several creative communities. Recognize that support comes in many forms and explore with your client what might work best for them. Do they

need peers? Professional contacts? Help applying for an artist's residency?

2. Be aware that your client may be dealing with the repercussions of being part of unsupportive or even toxic communities in the past. Help them understand that if a community does not feel like a good fit, it's time to move on – and also that past negative experiences don't mean they can't find a truly nurturing community.

3. Your client may come to you with conflicting advice or feedback they've received from communities they are in. They may need guidance on sorting through it to parse what is valuable and right for them. Through careful questions, you can guide them out of the feelings of overwhelm and confusion to a place where they feel empowered to make decisions about their work.

 ## About the Author

Jana Van der Veer is a writer and book coach at Set Your Muse on Fire, where she helps writers finally finish the book of their dreams. She also runs courses and programs to support women creatives in all stages of their careers. She has an MFA in creative writing from Lesley University and is an Author Accelerator–certified book coach as well as a certified creativity coach. Find her at www.setyourmuseonfire.com.

The Value of Support   **14**

Lisa Tener

It was during a retreat at the Kripalu Yoga Retreat Center, taught by this volume's co-editor Eric Maisel, that I became unblocked, books began to pour out of me and I was able to complete them after more than 15 years of unfinished and abandoned projects.

I'd been coaching aspiring authors to get their books and book proposals written, editing their work and teaching about book and proposal writing at Harvard Medical School's CME course on writing and publishing books for more than a dozen years. My clients had great success with writing award-winning books, negotiating five- and six-figure books deals and receiving national publicity from the *New York Times* to *Good Morning America* and beyond.

I felt proud of my coaching work but disappointed in myself as a creator. I started books – on my own or with colleagues. Yet I usually lost my passion for the project long before a first draft. I hadn't published a book of my own in over a decade.

Eric Maisel's workshop changed all that. Eric taught me why we procrastinate and how to combat the anxiety behind procrastination. His generous encouragement and the prolific writing I experienced shifted my belief in myself and my projects. I realized that I needed support in the form of:

- Understanding what blocked me and how to get unblocked
- The safe, inspiring and powerful creative container the retreat provided
- The confidence that prolific writing returned to me and the joyful state that prompted more and more writing
- Tools to stay engaged, committed and prolific

External support includes cultivating an environment conducive to our creative work and having people in our lives who support us – friends, colleagues, online groups, teachers, coaches, mentors, etc.

DOI: 10.4324/9781003351344-14

The Muse as Internal Creative Support

The other game changer was my inner muse. I lead my clients through a creative visualization exercise I call "Meet Your Muse," during which they gather their questions and then I guide them through imagining a journey to their muse, deep in the forest. In this sacred space, we ask the clients' inner muse questions: how to fully commit to their creative work, what direction to take, why X isn't working, how to make their creative habits more effective, how to transform insecurity and feelings of not being worthy into a sense of worth and confidence, etc. Then we ask, "What else does the muse want us to know?"

I needed to do that exercise myself!

While teaching a workshop on book writing for the International Coaching Federation of New England, I stayed for the second presentation of the day, given by Tama Kieves. Within a few minutes, I knew that she could help me connect with my muse. I taught Tama the "Meet Your Muse" exercise and asked her to lead me through it. We do that exercise every time I call her and now I have the beautiful connection with my muse that I longed for.

Why couldn't I do that exercise alone? It helps to have another person witness and hold space for the experience. If I just travel into la-la land with my muse, I easily forget my questions, or else I find it hard to go deep, knowing I also need to facilitate the questions myself. With a guide, I can go deep while Tama keeps me focused. Some people can easily internalize that connection and get clarity through journaling or other means. For me, the deep state from the guided visualization is key.

Creative Work Requires Support

The bottom line is that to get our creative work done, we need support. And that support means internal support (connection with our muse, as well as a practice that consistently supports our creative activity) and external support (community, environment, a coach, a course, a creative partner).

What follows is some brief guidance for getting and offering support, along with five simple – and brilliant – questions I learned from coach Mitch Feinberg to help you (and your clients) stay on track to complete creative work. I have used this easy-to-use, effective system for accountability in my classes for over a decade.

Guidelines for Giving and Receiving Support

You can start by simply asking, "What are my biggest creative challenges? Where am I getting stuck?" Some possibilities include:

- Ineffective habits and mindset
- A lack of connection with my creative source
- Not enough accountability, commitment and completion
- Self-doubt, feeling unworthy, questioning whether people want what I have to offer, or whether it will be good enough
- Not sure what to write/create
- A lack of clarity of direction
- Too many project ideas
- Overwhelm
- Other challenges

Once you identify the challenges, consider which environments and types of support best fit those needs. Possibilities include:

- Checking in with an accountability partner
- Direct guidance, insights, coaching and accountability with a coach or mentor
- A course, in person or online
- An online or in-person community
- A breakthrough, such as a shift in mind frame and habits

For help in choosing a project or direction, developing a structure, or experiencing a breakthrough, you may just need one or more sessions. For accountability, you may need an ongoing relationship. Assess which types of support will best work for you by keeping in mind the depth of the issue, the time commitment involved and your budget.

The Five Questions

Mitch's five questions can be asked daily or weekly:

1. What did I commit to?
2. What did I actually do?
3. What worked?
4. What didn't work?
5. What's next? (This becomes your commitment for the coming week or whatever time period you designate.)

What's so brilliant about Mitch's system is that the answers to numbers three and four inform number five. You do more of what worked, problem solve what didn't work and fine-tune your plans to make it work more smoothly.

For example, let's say that you scheduled time in your calendar for your creative project. It worked most days, but it didn't work on the day your mom surprised you by dropping in unannounced. "What's next?" might be letting your mom know that she needs to make plans with you by phone, or it might be letting her know your writing schedule and that you're not available during those times.

A Burned-Out Therapist Finds His Spark

A therapist in my Bring Your Book to Life® program hadn't written all week. Upon checking in, he shared his plans to write the following week. What would be different, though? We examined what didn't work and why. He planned to write on weekends, only to find himself burned out from his weekly caseload and unable to create. I suggested that he energize and recharge before writing – a walk in nature, meditation, yoga. He said listening to music rejuvenated him. The following class, after scheduling music time before each writing session, he reported a creatively rich weekend.

Key to making this system work – particularly when two people serve as each other's accountability partners – is a quick, streamlined process. You're not chatting on the call; you're saving your time and energy for creative work and neither person is coaching the other. The accountability partner simply asks the five questions and then listens for the answer. The other person looks inward to identify what didn't work, why and how to prevent the problem in the future. If the partner feels strongly that their ideas could be of help, they can wait until the end of the exercise and ask, "I have an idea; would you like to hear it?"

   Three Tips for Creatives

1. Find an accountability partner and together ask the five questions weekly.
2. If looking for a course or coach, be clear what kind of support you want and need. Is it accountability? Technique? Coaching for a

breakthrough? Interview the coach and make sure the solution fits the problems you are encountering.

3. Practice gratitude. As with all relationships, as you nurture your relationship with your creative muse, it deepens. Don't beat your muse up when you've only produced half the number of pages you planned. Celebrate the five pages you did write or the time you set aside for creative pursuits.

 Three Tips for Coaches

1. To help client get the support they need, determine how the client currently receives internal support (creative connection) and external support (community, coaching). Explore what type of support is missing and needed: for example, skills or habits they need to learn, an accountability system, clarity on artistic direction, getting unblocked, getting their work out into the world, etc.

2. To help clients connect to their inner muse, after talking through a possible creative direction, invite your clients to connect with their inner muse, whether through a guided visualization or some other means and have them confirm the creative choices you've discussed. Help them find various ways to consult – and develop a relationship with – their muse, such as journaling (for example, a dialogue with the muse).

3. To help your clients see what they're doing right, celebrating wins helps build confidence. If we focus only on what's not working, we risk decreased confidence, reduced commitment and loss of enthusiasm.

   With strong external and internal support, the foundation is in place for a consistent creative habit to help you – and your creative clients – complete projects and get them out into the world.

About the Author

Lisa Tener is an award-winning author, book writing and publishing coach and speaker. Her recent book, *The Joy of Writing Journal: Spark Your Creativity in 8 Minutes a Day*, won the 2022 Nautilus Book Award and Independent Publisher Award (IPPY). Lisa received the Stevie Award for Coach/Mentor and has helped thousands of writers tap into their creativity and publish. Her clients have signed five- and six-figure book deals with Hachette, Random House and other top publishers. Lisa has been quoted in the *New York Times*, *Boston Globe* and *Vice* and has appeared on national and local TV, including PBS. Learn more at LisaTener.com.

Shaping Routines That Work

15

Anne Carley

Do you rebel at the thought of routines? Do you prefer to be unencumbered during the creative time that's available? That was me, for most of my life. I'm finding, however, a new way to use routines to help me complete creative projects. Although most of my creative work these days involves writing, the following ideas can adapt to other forms of creative expression, too.

What Is the Relationship of a Habit to a Routine?

Opinions vary. For our purposes here, a habit is an ingrained behavior that we do unthinkingly. A routine is a repeated behavior or sequence of linked behaviors that may or may not be habitual.

I have routines, for example, that occur during the November-December holiday season. I don't repeat them often enough for them to be habitual and yet I am comforted each year when it comes time to revisit them. Other routines, like caring for my teeth, are ingrained daily habits. I cultivate other daily routine behaviors, like journaling and meditation and sometimes miss a day.

When I considered my creative routines, I was initially discouraged. My behavior all looked pretty basic. Sit with notebook or laptop. Draft sentences. Pause. Repeat. Where could I begin to institute a routine? Then the deeper insight revealed itself: I was already observing routines!

Our neurological preference is for unexamined living. Changing habits and routines is so hard to do because unthinking behavior saves a lot of effort and

DOI: 10.4324/9781003351344-15

energy and protects us from unexpected harm. I picture my brain's brawny enforcers glaring at me, their thickly muscled forearms crossed belligerently, when I consider an alteration to my usual behavior.

When is it worth it to struggle against those enforcers? What makes me dedicate myself to changing an unexamined, comfortable state? It does require dedication, over a period of weeks, months and even years. A whim isn't strong enough to go up against those enforcers and succeed.

We need to rally our determination and consistent effort if we want to intervene and create a new creative routine, displacing what's been chugging along in the background just fine, thank you.

Three Unexamined Routines

In its unceasing efforts to conserve energy and protect me from harm, my brain had quietly created routines – behind my back, so to speak. And once I began examining those routines, I could see they might be efficient for my brain, but some of them weren't serving me or my creative purposes. In fact, they were moving the finish line further and further away.

Distraction: *"Squirrel!"* Like Dug the dog in the movie *Up*, I am open to sudden distractions, especially when I'm avoiding finishing a project. *OMG I just remembered that email I promised someone this afternoon! Those towels aren't going to wash themselves! I have a great idea for my next blog – I'll just make a few notes!* I experience some excitement, do some minor unrelated tasks and make no progress.

Numbing: If a project and I are at odds and I don't know how to get it done, another fallback routine behavior is checking out my news feed on Twitter. Doomscrolling takes me away, absorbs some of my attention as well as a chunk of my time and leaves me listless and unmotivated, no closer to a conclusion.

Overworking: This routine is sneaky. While actively working on completing a project, I keep going and going. I go longer than I have the energy to remain effective. When I do stop, it's at a random place. I also associate a worn-out feeling, perhaps even dread, with my next visit to the incomplete project.

All three of those routines resulted in a loss of focused energy. They had the power to derail me so much that I forgot what I intended to do. And, of course, the projects didn't get finished.

I'm now on a mission to craft energy-efficient routines that also align with my creative purposes and permit me to get all the way to DONE.

Here are things I have learned that are helpful to establish in order to get things done.

Calm: An important routine to establish, if you don't already have one, is a calming practice. To replace the buzzing, frantic, disorganized vibe that derails the creative process, find a reliable way to shift to a slower, more focused mode that permits the creative parts of the brain to come back online. This is how to gather your energies to undertake the final effort to complete a major project.

Downtime: Avoid the trap of assuming that all your creative time must be spent in production mode. We differ from each other and we also change over time, so be aware of your current needs. Close to the end of a project, rushing isn't always wise. Sometimes the best work arrives after a pause for reflection.

Reward: Consider the value of a routine to mark, track and thereby reward progress. Each little gift to the brain's reward center cheers us up and makes us want to return for more. What's a good reward? It can be a cup of tea, a checkmark on a progress chart, or a five-minute exercise "snack." No need to wait for the end. Chunk down a larger project and celebrate the successful completion of sub-parts along the way to the finish line.

My Three Routines: An Update

Of my three unexamined routines, I began with limiting my social media time because it was the least nuanced and easiest to track. That new routine required at least a month to get solidly entrenched. Next came the distraction-busting statement of my minimum expectation for each work session. That took me about six weeks to implement reliably.

Then I began the ongoing process of checking in with myself during a productive session so that I end it before I'm too depleted and at a stopping point I'm eager to revisit.

Distraction (Squirrel!): Before starting a work session, I do purposeful breathing and say out loud my minimum expectation – measured in minutes or words or something else – toward completing a specified project during that session. I find I often exceed my minimum, which I intentionally set on the low side, as I stick to my stated purpose. One completed session after the next adds up to a satisfactorily concluded project.

Numbing (Twitter): I allocate certain times of day and days of the week to visit Twitter. I've extended these limits to other social media as well because they all exert the same energy-zapping effect. I stay calmer when writing and, my projects get completed quicker now.

Overworking (Forgetting to Stop): When I sit down to write, I commit to stopping at a place I'll be eager to see again. I am also learning to check in with myself as I'm working. This allows me to discern when I'm sliding toward overdoing it and to stop before that happens. Taking a break feels like a reward, not defeat. I walk away happy about what I have done, looking forward to returning. This way, the project wraps up sooner and with more enjoyment along the way.

I'm seeing clear benefits to all three new routines. My brain's brawny enforcers have new routines to protect. They help me complete creative tasks more calmly and provide me lovely moments filled with the pleasures of accomplishment. These routines also clear out mental cobwebs while supporting focus and optimism. What's not to like?

Final Thoughts

Because our human brain will combine behaviors into routines, whether we like them or not, it makes sense to examine those routines and shape them to serve our purposes. When we do, we'll finish what we started and enjoy the process along the way.

Three Tips for Creatives

1. Have you begun a host of projects and only finished a few (or none)? Consider taking the time to sort through all your current projects and limit your focus to one and one alone. This way, you're more likely to finish it.
2. Is your big project boring you? It's possible you're operating under some stale priorities. Step away from your workplace and get clear about what's important to you right now. Reset your to-dos and routines accordingly.
3. In a burst of resolve, do you want to completely rebuild your working routines before you finish the current project? Don't let your good intentions distract you. Changing one thing at a time is more likely to be effective. Commit to one new routine that will help you finish what you're working on. Later, shape another routine. And so on.

 Three Tips for Coaches

1. Is your client having trouble concentrating on the project they need to complete? Recommend a breathing routine to incorporate at crucial points during a work session.
2. Are your clients' concerns hijacking the completion of your own project? Put a compass image or object in plain view in your workspace. It can be coded – perhaps an object or photo that has deep meaning to you or elegantly printed text, reminding you of your specific purpose. Zero in on it whenever your resolve has wandered off course and get your project to completion.
3. Is your client mostly done with their main project and already off exploring new ideas? Now is a good time to shape a reliable routine for storing and retrieving those new ideas. When the client can trust that the new material will be at hand later, it'll be easier to complete the primary project.

About the Author

Anne Carley is a coach, editor, author and composer. Once she recognized that she could shape her own routines, she began enjoying writing more and got more projects done. Her handbook, *FLOAT • Becoming Unstuck for Writers* and the FLOAT Cards for Writers deck provide methods and interventions for writers and other creatives to shift out of stuckness and back into creative flow. Visit annecarleycreative.com for blog posts, articles and more about shaping your creative process.

Moving from Self-Doubt into Self-Leadership

16

Sharon Stratford

When I first met Chris, he was stuck in self-doubt, trapped in his head playing out worst-case scenarios, pestering himself with worries and negative thoughts and stirred up by churning emotions. Three months earlier, he had been sparking with energy and excitement after taking a life-changing leap into the unknown. He had resigned from his high-paying job to jump full time into his creativity, letting go of the structure, predictability and financial stability he had known. Chris was now free to build the stimulating life he wanted for himself, working full time on his ambitious artistic project.

The problem was that none of it was going according to plan. His intentions were bold. He wanted to write the content and produce the video for the story he was going to tell, but every day, he smothered his storyboard in details. Chris was great at generating detailed lists and notes. He knew how to do that. He didn't know how to translate those details into storytelling. The difficulty and importance of the task overwhelmed him. After three months of overwhelm, he was trapped in the gap between his intentions and actions, riding the storm that many creators struggling with completion confront. He found himself taking a daily beating from his inner critic. It was time to shift from self-doubt into self-leadership, but first, Chris had to understand what he was up against.

Our habits, beliefs and personalities are complex characters that shape how we think, feel and act. We need to learn their stories and the voice that tells them through self-reflection and journaling. Switch off your autopilot. Connect to your critical and creative thinking. Invite curiosity in and express who you are in writing. Reflect on your experiences so that you can make

DOI: 10.4324/9781003351344-16

sense of yourself. If you want to complete your ambitious creative project, you have to learn to master these complex characters. Find the will to spend time in self-reflection and journal writing every day so that you can navigate this tangle of teachers and tricksters.

Deciding to actively learn about ourselves allows us to see our dynamic personality in action. We hold within us a tension of tendencies that can drive or drain our energy and efforts. In tough times, we want our primary preferences to take the lead because they are easy for us. We can trigger these parts of our personality naturally and we can hang out with them for a long time because we've practiced them for years. Caught in overwhelm, we can put them in the driver's seat and work them until they are exhausted.

Then, out of the shadows, come those awkward, edgy parts of our personality – those aspects of ourselves that we don't express as much because they sit outside our comfort zone. We need them. Relying solely on the preferred parts of our personality puts us off balance and cuts us off from trying new thoughts, feelings, or actions that will get us moving and get our projects across the finish line. When we are being smacked by self-doubt and crippled by old patterns of behavior that don't serve us, we need to go into the shadows and meet our potential there.

Taking a deep dive into his personality, we could see that Chris relied on past experience to inform and guide him. His personality wanted accurate details and a logical plan to get things done. Working independently on his creative project without the structure and predictability of his previous working life was a new experience. There was no proven method to give him a clear plan or logical solution, which sparked his imagination to see all the worst possible outcomes. He was swamped by a sense of personal failure and defeat.

Chris had to power up his potential. If he could challenge his personality to get out of its comfort zone by trying some new thoughts and actions, he might become his own daring leader instead of surrendering to self-doubt. He had been telling himself every day that failure was not an option . . . but what if he was wrong? What if he replaced that thought with *Failure is an option*. He constantly demanded perfection from himself and when his competence was called into question, he would abandon his project to go and do something that he was good at. What if he dared himself to be a student instead of an expert?

We agreed to use his love of exercise to prime his brain and body for the creative work to follow. So, after exercising every morning, Chris committed to three to four hours of work on his creative project and challenged himself to become a beginner, open to making mistakes and messes. We created a safe environment for his imagination to enjoy some serious play through crafted experiments and self-reflection. When we experiment, there is no right or wrong, better or worse – only curiosity and lessons learned.

We called on his creativity and experience to give his project a name, vision, values and a new story to champion. After six weeks of cheerleading and challenges, devotion and discipline, his design business came to life, powered by values of stimulation, purpose, flow, creativity and fun. The significance Chris gave to each value inspired his vision to "design meaningful learning experiences that make a difference for people through emotional connection, storytelling and innovation."

While doing the values work, we discovered a deeply buried nugget of self-deception. Chris believed he wasn't culturally competent to write these stories or share them with others. We busted this inherited belief by establishing Chris as the editor of this limiting story. By paying attention to his internal narrator, confronting the origins of this fiction and challenging its truth, he was able to craft and champion the power of a new story. He was in the magic zone. He had produced his first video, was starting on his second and had teamed up with a new business partner. The storm he had been riding was quietly passing by.

Stories can predict the future through reasoning, intuition, mischief making, or magic. Our clients will live whatever story they are telling. If they are getting in their own way, help them rewrite the narrative by reminding them that they control the context, the conflict and the conclusion for each chapter.

It's easy to surrender to our autopilot and let old, familiar habits and beliefs take charge while we curl up, cozy in our comfort zone, hanging out with those trusted parts of our personality that we know and like so much. Here, we feel competent and know what to expect. There is little or no risk, few challenges and no magic. Like a warm bath, a comfort zone can be welcoming and relaxing – a retreat when we need to rest and recharge – but a warm bath can grow cold if we stay in it too long!

Working with Chris made me realize that I had abandoned my own ambitions and creative process, so I challenged myself to take the adventure with him. By committing to every action I asked of him, I discovered my own nugget of self-deception. My story was based on a powerful inherited belief that "work isn't fun, creative, or playful," and so I had stuffed my day full of things I *should* do instead of things I *loved* to do. I had drained all the motivation out of my creative work by living by someone else's rule book. Once I was back in the magic zone of self-direction, I could decide my identity and my destiny and lead myself to live that experience.

Three Tips for Creatives

1. Show up for yourself every day to practice the art of self-reflection and writing. Open up a conversation between your thoughts, emotions and actions. Go into the shadows and discover those awkward, edgy parts of your personality. Get to know these dynamic characters and claim your right to govern them. Intentionally direct yourself to take consistent, meaningful action to achieve your ambitious project.
2. Promote your values to the position of five-star leaders. If you form a purposeful connection with these allies and advisors, they can reshape self-doubt into self-leadership. Invest in them and they will strengthen your resilience and your relationship with completion.
3. We give meaning to our experiences, our beliefs and our identity and these giants shape our lives. We can push these giants in a new direction because we create them. Champion the power of your story. If changing your narrative will enable you to finish your creative project – then rewrite it. Every day, experiment with one new thought and/or one new action to develop your writing style.

Three Tips for Coaches

1. Always be curious about that mysterious space between intentions and actions. We are not the experts here – our clients are the way finders in this wilderness – and we are their students. Spark their self-knowledge and stimulate their thinking with big questions like:

   - Why does this matter to you?
   - What beliefs are stopping you from finishing?
   - Do you have clear values or principles guiding you?
   - How is your personality getting in your way?
   - What simple step can you take today to jump into action?

2. Too many clients live with the conflict between what they want to do and what they believe they can do. It's important to help them bust inherited beliefs that don't serve them and resolve values that are in conflict with one another.

3. Take your clients through a values exercise that has personal meaning. Support them to identify these guides and define their essence.

 ## About the Author

Sharon Stratford is a writer, creativity coach and personality navigator. She has qualifications in coaching, personality dynamics, writing and adult teaching. Madly in love with ambitious, creative projects and the sparkling attraction of starting something new, she has struggled to get to the finish line or call something completed. With over 15 years of coaching and personal experience, she firmly believes in the vitality of creativity and is always learning how to nurture it constructively. For her, that means daily creative work and disciplined self-leadership to achieve completion.

How Grace, Gratitude and Generosity Can Help Us Find the Path Forward

17

Michele Blackwell

Often, creative projects don't go as planned. We start in a flurry of creative inspiration but get lost midway. It can be frustrating to find ourselves neck deep in a project we started with enthusiasm and suddenly feel adrift, like a swimmer who dives excitedly into the ocean and comes up for air, only to discover that she is uncomfortably far from shore. Anxiety builds and can be further exacerbated by an approaching deadline.

This chapter offers three tools to shift our mindset when we find ourselves stuck – grace, gratitude and generosity. They can be beneficial in all aspects of our lives but can be especially helpful when we need to reframe our creative process mid-project.

We begin with high expectations. How can we not? In those flashes of imagination that spurred us to start, we have a bright vision of what we want to manifest. We dive in. But as we try to realize that vision, it can feel like we are being tossed about in a tumultuous ocean.

When I was studying design at UCLA, I had a habit of starting my critique presentations with an explanation of what wasn't working with my project. An instructor suggested I stop doing that. "What you see in your mind is perfect," he said. "Nothing you create is going to be as good as your vision. But here's the thing – only you can see what's in your mind's eye. The rest of us see just the work. And to us, it may be beautiful."

Suddenly I questioned my thoughts about my creative work. But now I saw it. The work existed, independent of my feelings about it. I realized

DOI: 10.4324/9781003351344-17

I could be attached to my vision of the work, accept it and also accept the output without condemnation. This is grace.

A young singer/songwriter, Nadia, reached out for help. She was working on songs for her first solo record. Coming from a family of successful musicians, she grew up in the recording industry. Now she was attempting to make her mark, but the bridge of one song had her stuck. To complicate matters, her father kept checking to see how she was coming along. She told him everything was fine, but inwardly, she was measuring her ability to complete this song against her father's accomplishments. Sensing she was struggling, he kept insisting she needed help, but Nadia was determined to do it on her own. She began a downward spiral of negative self-talk and soon found herself unable to make any progress at all.

Nadia and I worked with the concept of grace. She had set an extremely high bar for herself, based on the expectations of her family and her desire to prove that she could match their achievements.

I reminded her that she was working on four songs. Having one that wasn't coming together didn't seem so terrible if she considered how much she was creating. I suggested she pause on the one that wasn't working.

As she eased up on herself, she began to relax. Eventually, the bridge for the song she was struggling with came to her.

Grace is a radical acceptance of where you are in your creative project AND how you feel about where you are.

Grace separates reality from judgment. It's stepping back and taking a breath. You put the work down, pause and return to it later, perhaps with a new perspective.

A telltale sign that we have not given ourselves grace is negative self-talk. It's one thing to find ourselves blocked. It's quite another to begin barraging ourselves with disempowering statements. Negative self-talk is like trying to swim with an anchor tied around our necks. They weigh us down. The work is already turbulent enough without the added weight of our hypercritical selves pulling us under.

Offering ourselves grace is more than just casting off the self-doubt anchors; it is a lifesaving buoy to rest upon when things get too choppy. Instead of trying to calm the sea, we are finding a safe place to regain our strength.

To cultivate grace, start where you are. Deconstruct the creative process. If you are a painter, grab a brush, mix some colors and make random brushstrokes. Let yourself feel the flow that ignites when paint, brush and canvas merge. Don't try to create anything in particular.

A writer might experiment with alliteration just to put words onto the page. How many variations of "She sells seashells by the seashore" can you create? Dive in with a sense of improvisation. Have fun simply playing with words.

Warm-up exercises work because they signal the brain to get into flow. They bypass the inner critic "security guard" that wants everything to be perfect. They make space. It's just practicing, but practice is *everything*.

Gratitude is discovering the good in your unfinished work. There is beauty inherent in your work in progress. Find it. Appreciate it.

The plot of your screenplay feels contrived, but your dialogue is pithy. The lyrics of that last verse of your song may not resonate, but the bridge is magical. Look for what's right and how you might expand those qualities. Don't just notice what's working; honor it. Your efforts thus far are evidence of your talent and ability. It's important to acknowledge that. Gratitude for what you have made coaxes you gently back into possibility.

Generosity is honoring your talent and conviction by giving yourself what you need to feel safe, appreciated and supported in your work.

Another client, Sandra, was stuck with her screenplay. She had completed the first draft, but when it came to doing revisions, she couldn't focus. She told me her inner child was "being a spoiled brat" who demanded ice cream every time she sat down to work. As hard as she tried, Sandra found herself continually pulled out of her chair by all manner of distractions, including the sound of the ice cream truck passing through her neighborhood each day.

I asked her, "Why can't your inner child have some ice cream?"

She thought for a moment and replied, "She can have ice cream after we do the work."

"Why can't she have the ice cream beforehand?" She didn't have an answer. "What do you think your inner child wants?"

Sandra realized ice cream represented comfort. She concluded that her inner child really wanted attention. "Why do you think your inner child needs this attention just as you sit down to work?"

"Because that part is scary," she said.

Sandra's dilemma is common among writers. They worry that they will ruin their work when they attempt to refine it. The first draft is easy. The revision is hell.

"What if you could give yourself comfort before you start?"

Sandra agreed to try. She happily reported later that she had found ways to ease herself into the work with small rewards. Who says you can't start with dessert and finish the evening with steak? If having dessert first is what gets you to the table, then do that.

Three Tips for Creatives

1. Offer yourself grace. If you are stuck, acknowledge it and let it be okay. Pause without melodrama or negative self-talk.
2. Find gratitude for how far you've come. Find ten things about your project in progress for which you are grateful.
3. Be generous. Support yourself. Ask "What do I need to keep going or restart?" Indulge a little to congratulate yourself on what you've done thus far. Give yourself the ice cream.

Three Tips for Coaches

1. When our clients are stuck, they can be incredibly hard on themselves. Offer them grace, hold space for them and affirm that it is okay to be right where they are. To help clients separate what is happening with their creative process from how they feel about it, you might ask them to state where they are with the project as a percentage of completion. Ask "How do you feel about being __% done with your project?" This can break the connection between what is and their judgment of it.
2. Prompting clients to celebrate how far they have come can help them find gratitude for their creative projects. Have your client place their current project on a wall. Have them place a large sheet of newsprint next to it and write out everything that is going right with the project. Ask them to leave it on the wall for at least two days, adding only what is working to the list. Check in during your next session to see what they've discovered.
3. Encouraging clients to build "little rewards" into their creative practice can aid them in becoming more generous with themselves. Ask "How can we make your practice more fun? In what ways can you be more giving to yourself? What support might you need from others to keep moving forward?"

Adding the elements of grace, gratitude and generosity to the creative practice offers self-care, validation and self-reward. We can use these mind-shift tools to find compassion and presence, wherever we are in the process of our projects. Grace is acknowledgement and acceptance of where we are. It allows us to suspend judgment, which, in turn, can ease creative anxiety. Gratitude refocuses us on the parts of the project that are working, which aids in returning to a state of flow. Generosity leads us to discover what support we need to fortify ourselves and make our creative practice more joyful. Together, they help us avoid negativity spirals when faced with waves of uncertainty, find the stamina to finish and build resilience for future projects.

 ## About the Author

Michele Blackwell is a photographer, filmmaker, designer and coach. She has a film degree from the University of Miami, an MBA from Pepperdine University and advanced professional certificates from UCLA in producing and screenwriting. As a coach, she works with entrepreneurs looking to build sustainable businesses from their creative endeavors. Learn more at www.mabmultimedia.com.

The Power of a Secular Shabbat Practice

18

Helen L. Conway

Jake was sick of his book. Three years ago, he had committed to writing a meticulously researched historical novel. He let go of some of his business consulting work to free up time for a daily writing habit. He invested vacation time and money to travel to his book's location and interview experts on the era. For a long time, his project gave him great joy and purpose. Now, however, he was stuck.

The book felt never ending. The more he worked, the more options he had to grapple with and the less able he was to make decisions. His process had dwindled from a joyous flow of words each day to hours of painful editing. He felt he was just moving paragraphs around endlessly. The book was not bad, far from it – members of his writers' group had praised his writing. It was just that he couldn't seem to get it to the endpoint. He couldn't find a way to tie the strands of the plot together. He began to tell himself that he didn't have what it took, that he was only good for the play part at the beginning of the process, not for the "real work" of being an author.

He hoped coaching would give him productivity techniques to help him get more out of his writing sessions and enable him to "push through hard until the end." Looking at his work habits, however, showed that he was dedicated, he was working regular hours and producing a respectable word count or editing a fair number of pages. He wasn't, however, finding the answer to his plotting problem. And without that, he would never complete the book.

I suggested a counterintuitive move. I invited him to stop working and to take a regular secular Shabbat from his work.

Shabbat (plural: Shabbatot) is a Jewish concept but was carried over into Christianity as "sabbath". The word means "cessation" in Hebrew. On one day in every seven, work stops. This is where we get the idea of a sabbatical,

DOI: 10.4324/9781003351344-18

the extended period off written into many work contracts, often at a seven-year interval. It is closely tied to the stories previous generations have told to explain how the world was created. However, no religious affiliation is needed to reap the benefit of a secular Shabbat.

Of course, to cease work, you first must know what constitutes work. The ancient Jewish texts set out 39 different acts, which fall into four classes of activity. They all relate to creation. On Shabbat, one refrains from creating food, shelter, or clothing and, interestingly, from writing. Art forms are as vital to our well-being as our physical needs and yet the Shabbat suggests we take a break from attending to all of them once every week.

Why would you take a day off, only to deny yourself the joy of creativity? Well, first, a secular Shabbat is not about being miserable and restricted. The exact opposite. The idea is that you have a complete change and embrace the other forms of joy in life you may have set aside to commit to your creative project. No one starves on Shabbat. Food is prepared in advance and the usual chores are set aside to allow time to enjoy a special meal. Try the same thing on a secular Shabbat. Get your desk or studio tidied up and enjoy time with family, walk in the woods, or go to the theatre. Do whatever fills you up and makes you smile. Get your head up from the keyboard and take in the world. Creativity requires that we are full of experiences so that we can use them in our creative work.

One aspect of a secular Shabbat is that it allows us to restore ourselves physically. Stepping away from the keyboard or easel allows us to use our body differently, resting tired, overused muscles. It allows us to rest and get exercise, to take our stinging eyes away from our screens. A short period of absence allows us to miss our work, to see it again as enticing and beguiling.

So much of the quality of creative work is about the differences that the creator places within it. A good novel has characters who think and talk differently to each other. Tension in the plot depends on the conflict arising when one character wants something different from another. In a painting, there may be differences in color values, shapes and quality of lines to draw the viewer's attention. As humans, we thrive on differences and find them exciting. A secular Shabbat allows you to create a difference in pace and activity within your own creative life.

A secular Shabbat also allows us to access our unconscious. An important part of a secular Shabbat is that we stop even thinking about our creative projects. Jake was skeptical about the idea of a Shabbat but desperate enough to complete the book that he decided to try spending every Sunday not writing. The first couple of weeks, he took the opportunity to go for a run instead. He found the exercise did give him more energy for his writing. However, he reported back that as he pounded the trail, he ended up pondering whether he should kill his main character off and came back just as stuck.

Allowing our project to constantly occupy every waking thought means we get stuck in our conscious minds. In turn, that prevents us from fully experiencing the creative process. Graham Wallas, in his book *The Art of Thought*, as long ago as 1926 identified that the four key stages of creativity were preparation, incubation, illumination and validation. The first and the last we do consciously; the illumination is the experience we have when an idea or solution appears to us. That, however, can't happen unless we incubate the problem and that happens in our unconscious. As Wallas explained, "It is desirable not only that there should be an interval free from conscious thought on the particular problem but also that the interval should be so spent that nothing should interfere with the free working of the unconscious."

Jake decided to set out on his run the next week with a sports podcast on to take his mind away from his writing. The next week, it snowed and he chose instead to spend his time playing games with his children. Soon he found that he was training himself to "leave the book aside," and yet when he came back to it, he felt refreshed and had a clearer idea of how to get it toward completion.

> After a while, he hit on another benefit of a secular Shabbat. "I think deep down I was afraid to let go," he said.I'd put so much time into this and it gave me my longed-for identity as a writer. But I didn't have any ideas yet for a second book. The idea of completing this one made me afraid I'd never be able to start again. Then who would I be?

Practicing stopping and starting again in a small way gave him the confidence to complete his book, knowing that even if there was a short period before his new idea came to him, the sky would not fall in. He began to see that a buffer zone between projects was akin to a sabbatical and held a real benefit. A secular Shabbat can help us trust in the fact that the "muse" or "inspiration" (or whatever word you use to describe that mysterious partnership that seems to happen in creativity) will not abandon us if we rest awhile.

Jake completed his novel and to celebrate, he took his family on a special vacation. Exploring Rome with a guide, he heard a little-known historical story that inspired his second novel. He is now writing a third and has maintained his weekly secular Shabbat. Every seven months, he takes a short trip to a place with an interesting history. "Not to formally research," he says.

> I always go to somewhere that has nothing to do with the book I am working on. I even spent a weekend at a medieval jousting festival! It's

just my time to indulge in being that history nerd I was as a kid so that my enthusiasm is always topped up and shows through in my novels. I'm happy to complete work because I'm always full of ideas for the next one!

Three Tips for Creatives

1. Decide for yourself what counts as "work" for your project. What will you cease doing on your sabbatical?
2. Then think about setting a "fence" around these activities. What might cause you to slip into them accidentally? Are there secondary activities that are best not done because they will tempt you back to your project? Or choices you can make that will help you not to do so?
3. Don't view your sabbatical as an endurance or a necessary evil. This is a holiday you get every week, a celebration of your creativity. Consider how you will bring joy, connection and indulgence into your day off.

Three Tips for Coaches

1. Explore with the client's internalized messages about work. Do they believe it must all be an endless, hard slog? Can they adjust their mindset so that work also incorporates cessation?
2. If clients are reluctant to let go, explore what it is they believe they are holding on to. What are they afraid of if they stop?
3. Introduce clients to meditation techniques to help them learn and practice how to let unwanted thoughts about their work drift away without latching on to them.

About the Author

Helen L. Conway is an internationally exhibited artist with work in collections on four continents. She is also a published author, a creativity coach and a former judge. As well as qualifications in law and criminology, she holds an MA in writing studies from the University of Lancaster, a diploma in personal performance coaching and a PG certification in psychosynthesis and leadership coaching from Middlesex University. She specializes in helping artists, writers and lawyers think differently so they can create the life they wish to lead. Visit www.helenconway.com.

When the End Is Near **19**

Creative Finishing

Jacqui Beck

As we near completion of a creative project, it can be challenging and disheartening if we discover that it is not working in some way. The idea of having to reenter the work to make changes feels daunting. Also, we've been inside the work for so long that it can be hard to step back and truly see it.

This chapter presents some ways to explore creative ideas on how to work with an almost-finished project in order to enhance it and find a real sense of completion. It's never too late to breathe new life into a creative work.

The tools presented in this chapter can be used to assess what needs to be changed, as well as to figure out how to make those changes.

Altering a project at the final stages can be tricky; take care to stay within the voice of the piece and to work from a creative space. Though finishing is the focus here, the practices offered can be used at any stage of the creative process.

Remember to focus on yourself first. Taking care of yourself will help you work from a place of inner stability and resourcefulness. And remember that there is a delicate balance between honest, caring assessment and perfectionism. Finishing a project is difficult for most of us. It can be terrifying to declare a work completed because NOTHING is ever perfect. One of my painting teachers, Skip Lawrence, says that a painting is finished when we are 87% satisfied. Imagine that!

Isabel and Perfectionism

A new client came to me for coaching to work specifically on finishing. I'll call her Isabel. She said that initially, she would work on a painting in an

DOI: 10.4324/9781003351344-19

open and connected way and would be very happy with it, but as she was getting close to being finished, she'd start to get quite critical of her work. She would cover up parts she later regretted losing and would add details that were unnecessary.

As we worked on this, she realized that it was hard for her to declare any work finished. To her, that meant it was supposed to be perfect and she knew in her heart that it wasn't. We talked about this and Isabel gradually came to ease up on her beliefs about what we can expect of ourselves as beautifully imperfect human beings.

Over time, Isabel practiced making work that was imperfect. She played and made messes. She wrote supportive notes to herself and taped them all over the walls of her studio. She learned to let a piece rest for a while as she got close to finishing and would meet with other artists to look at work together to get support about deciding what a painting still needed (sometimes nothing). Gradually, she began to share more of her exciting and imperfect work.

Set Your Work Aside for a While

It can be helpful to let your work rest. Leave it alone for a period of time, then come back to it with renewed ears and eyes. One painter told me that she likes to surprise herself with an almost-finished painting. She will set it aside for a period of time, then hang it in a place she'll see easily. This gives her a fresh perspective and she will either have a sense that the painting really is finished, or something will jump out at her that clearly needs attention.

Incubation

This is one of our greatest creative tools. When we ask ourselves a question like "What does this painting need?" or "What do I need to do to improve the conversation between Jim and Lucinda in Chapter 13?" and then just leave it to our brain to chew on and mull over the question, our brain very often will come up with answers. Unlike setting work aside, in this case, we are purposefully asking our subconscious mind to work on a specific question or problem.

I use this technique myself with great results. The only real downside is that my insights often come at around 3:00 a.m. and I need to scribble them down before I forget. I can usually manage to read my handwriting in the morning.

Ask Yourself: What Does "Finished" Feel Like?

It can be difficult for anyone to "know" when an artistic piece is complete. I asked a number of visual artists and writers (including clients) this question and these were some of their responses:

- "There's an inner feeling of YES. It's a body sensation of contentment mixed with excitement."
- "It is like a sense that the painting releases me."
- "It feels like excitement, like my body is tingly and more alive."
- "It's a body feeling, almost euphoric – a sense that it's working."

Having a Conversation With Your Work – An Exercise

"What does my work need in order to be finished?" This isn't a question for your rational brain only. This exercise offers a way to access deeper or more subconscious resourcefulness. As with any good brainstorming, even weird and ridiculous ideas can be used to take you somewhere useful. This is an opportunity to get your creative juices flowing. Over the course of creating, there's a way that the work takes on a life of its own and you need to respect that and respond to it.

In this exercise, you'll have a "conversation" in which you ask yourself questions and then respond as your project. This may seem strange or even uncomfortable at first, but it can help you discover some useful information. You may want to take notes or record your conversation. Feel free to add your own questions or change any of the ones here to fit who you are and the piece you're working on.

Before You Begin

- Make sure that you have a private space and adequate time to delve deeply
- Get pen and paper and/or a recording device
- Center yourself and take some slow, deep breaths
- Hold an attitude of caring and curiosity, not judgment

Suggested Questions to Ask Your Work

- Is there anything you still need? Anything that isn't working?
- How can I make you even more interesting, beautiful, expressive, edgy, etc.?
- Have I overlooked something?
- What part of yourself do you like best? What part still feels a bit incomplete or off?
- Is there something you want to share/communicate/express that I haven't listened to or helped you with?
- Is there something you need that I don't yet understand or that I haven't been paying attention to?
- What do you need in order to feel complete?

I worked with a client who writes poetry. I'll call her Justine. She had a poem she'd worked on for months that she wanted to submit to a poetry journal. Justine really liked her poem but felt that it was missing something. As I explored this with her, she decided she would have a conversation with the poem.

We recorded her conversation so that she could focus on responding openly without having to remember what she'd said. The conversation went on for quite a while. Justine allowed for pauses but mostly just let the words flow. Some lovely and insightful bits of information emerged.

The core of what the poem shared with her was that it thought there was a lack of vulnerability and that she needed to share herself more deeply within the work. Justine then had to figure out how to reenter her poem to bring this out. She did this on her own after our session and began by again talking with her poem, asking it to help her see how to make these changes. She did a Save As and jumped in, promising herself that she would write whatever came to her and save editing for later.

 Three Tips for Creatives

1. Cultivate a sense of playfulness, messiness and wildness to discover ways to bring the excitement you have felt for your work along the way into the final stage.
2. Get curious. Ask yourself absurd or odd questions. For example: "Is it possible to end a piece of work with a question?" List ten ways to make a change you think is necessary.
3. Always go back to practicing self-care and reconnecting with yourself and your work.

Three Tips for Coaches

1. Even at this late stage, it is important to support your client to create with passion. You might say something like, "I get it that you're feeling overwhelmed and exhausted and yet, even at this late stage, it's important to work with your project from as genuine a place as you can. Let's look at some ways you can do that."
2. Even when a client recognizes a need to make some final changes, they can be afraid to reopen a nearly finished work. This is an opportunity to explore ways for them to understand their fear and reluctance and to find ways to move forward.
3. Explore with a client what "finished" feels like to them. This is beyond "I think this is finished." Share with them the necessity of assessing with their whole self, not just their rational brain.

    It's never too late to bring more life to our work. For a creative person or someone who supports people who create, the final stage of the work can be very challenging. To truly feel finished, we need to have a sense of YES about our work. There are many creative ways to figure out what areas are not quite finished, to discover what can be done and to find ways to integrate changes into the work. Using these creative approaches, our project can then come together in ways that enhance our experience and the project itself.

About the Author

Jacqui Beck is an artist, creativity coach and art educator. She has a master's degree in mental health counseling from the University of Victoria and has studied at Gage Academy of Art and with many nationally known artists. Jacqui has over 20 years of coaching experience and, as a practicing artist, has firsthand experience with the joys and struggles of the creative process. Visit www.jacquibeck.com.

Three Steps to Permanently Stop Procrastination

20

Steve Davit

Procrastination is one of our biggest enemies, stopping us from completing our creative projects. Every one of my clients and music friends has had several battles with procrastination and very few know how to win consistently.

In my own work, I've observed a formula that divides the projects that have overcome procrastination's allure from my unfinished projects still gathering dust on my hard drive.

In its simplest form, that formula is:

Specificity + Accountability + Deadlines = Completed Projects

When any one of those factors isn't there, my projects float in their liminal form, often remaining there forever.

When I bring all three together, I can go from start to finish without much friction.

Let's take a closer look at each step.

Step #1 – Specificity

As artists, we're often too vague with our work. We gravitate toward the ideas more than the execution – which leads to living in our heads and leaving the actual work for another day. Because of this, I find it useful to spend time answering these four questions when starting a new project:

1. What are you creating?
2. How are you creating it?

DOI: 10.4324/9781003351344-20

3.   Why are you creating it?
4.   What impact will it have on others?

The answer to the first question may seem obvious, but writing it down can focus your work on one specific idea.

The second question is a practical one. I like to answer it by breaking my project down into small chunks – something where I can "check the box" and know I am done. Examples of project chunks include writing one chapter of a book, recording a demo of a song, designing the artwork for an album, etc.

Questions three and four are also very useful for maintaining motivation from an existential perspective. I'll often look back at what I write as answers for these two questions when my progress on a project wanes, or I feel like my work has become aimless.

These answers may change throughout the course of the project, but as long as you know specifically what you need to do next, the project can continue moving toward the finish line.

Step #2 – Accountability

Accountability is when you are held responsible for the things you say you want to accomplish. It may come in the form of a friend, collaborator, editor, producer, mentor, coach, or someone in any number of roles. Having someone with whom you share your goals and progress will help ensure you finish your projects. And the more specific your goals are, the more helpful your accountability partner or group will be.

Step #3 – Deadlines

Without a clear endpoint, the perfectionist part of our minds will find all the little things that we could work on forever. The key to a good deadline is its being immediate enough to spur you into action but far enough away to allow ideas to simmer and evolve. Setting deadlines for the smaller chunks of your project helps keep you motivated. The deadlines also function as check-in points to see if you are on track.

Deadlines also work best when someone else can hold you accountable to them. Without my creativity coach, I tend to procrastinate and push back deadlines or never set them in the first place. But once I tell someone about a deadline or I promise a collaborator my part of the project by a certain date, I always find the time to finish.

Taken alone, specificity, accountability and deadlines are useful productivity tools. But when we combine them, they kick procrastination to the curb and make finishing creative projects a near inevitability.

Step #4 – Example: The Sleep Cycle Suite

My music project, the Sleep Cycle Suite, is a perfect example of how these things work together and how ignoring even one of them can derail the entire thing.

The project started out, as I'm sure many of you can relate to, as a desire to create with other humans after nearly 20 months of isolation. I had a lot of things I could do, so I answered the four questions to help me get more specific.

1. What am I creating?

   • An improvised score with several movements based on our sleep cycle

2. How am I creating it?

   • Write the score
   • Record the score
   • Mix the recording
   • Send to a mastering engineer
   • Release the recordings digitally

3. Why am I creating it?

   • To make music live with other musicians
   • Because I am fascinated by sleep

4. What impact will it have on others?

   • Get people to think about sleep and dreams in a new way
   • As a guide for collective improvisation for other musicians

Answering these questions gave me a map to get started, but the equation wasn't complete yet. Knowing I likely wouldn't get anything done without a proper deadline or people to hold me accountable, I booked a studio and hired musicians. If I didn't want to waste my time and money, I simply had to write the music and record it by the end of the studio session.

The writing and recording were easy, thanks to specificity, accountability and deadlines. Mixing is where things started to fall apart. I knew I wanted to "mix the recording" – but I couldn't specifically say what that meant or when I was done. I was also only accountable to myself and had no firm deadline to set a fire under me.

Procrastination was winning.

Once I set a goal to spend three to five more hours on the mix (specificity), told my mastering engineer when to expect the mix (accountability) and set a firm release date (deadline), I was able to let go of the little things and finish the mix.

Within a few weeks, I had the tracks mixed, mastered and released to the world.

Step #5 – Client Example: Mike's Demo

One of my clients – I'll call him Mike – has a strenuous full-time job and often feels like he doesn't have enough time or energy to actually complete his songs. I asked him to focus on just one meaningful project that he could complete within three weeks using my process. Here's what he came up with:

1. What am I creating?

   • A complete demo of a new song

2. How am I creating it?

   • Reflect on painful realizations about past relationships
   • Write the song on paper with my guitar
   • Record on my computer

3. Why am I creating it?

   • To turn my pain and my story into music as a form of recovery
   • To have an actual recording to share with others

4. What impact will it have on others?

   • To help other people who have gone through similar situations

I added additional accountability and specificity by inviting him to a feedback session in which some of my other clients share progress they've made on their projects.

Mike especially resonated with the group dynamic, telling me:

> I benefited from the accountability this process provided. I looked forward to sharing with the group at the end and it pushed me to get things done. It also allowed me to take the time to actually sit down and complete a song instead of writing little parts of multiple songs like I normally do. I really liked the focus and direction it provided.

We all struggle with procrastination and its alter ego, perfectionism. By applying specificity, accountability and deadlines to our projects, my clients and I have overcome their siren's song, leading to completed work. Together, we can win the war against procrastination with this magic formula by our side.

 Three Tips for Creatives

1. Get feedback on your work before it's finished – this can help you get specific with the chunk you want feedback on, provide someone to keep you accountable for the work and set a deadline to get the work ready for feedback. Writing out a list of questions will also help you direct the feedback to be as useful as possible.

2. Focus on either generating new ideas OR refining your current ideas. These processes use different parts of the brain and trying to do both at the same time or switching too rapidly will lead to writer's block or procrastination. New ideas work best when the analytical/judgmental part of our brain is turned off and editing works best when we can focus on refining what's there without cramming new ideas into the mix.

3. Go easy on yourself. We tend to overestimate what we'll make in a week or a month but underestimate what we'll make in a year or a decade. Your art will never see the light of day if you burn out before it's done, so make sure your process is sustainable for the long run.

Three Tips for Coaches

1. Weekly accountability groups will greatly improve your clients' output while creating a sense of community. They can also be a great starting point for artists unable to commit to one-on-one coaching.
2. Create your own creativity coach accountability group. I have been running one for almost a year now and it has helped me workshop ideas, given me new insights on particular problems and encouraged me to keep going when things got tough.
3. Use the "Yes and" game to brainstorm ideas with clients. Start with a problem and have your client think of a potential solution. You would then say, "Yes! What I like about that idea is ___, AND what about ___?" Your client would then say the same thing to you – and back and forth you go for as long as needed. This works especially well in group coaching, as it allows for more perspectives.

 ### About the Author

Steve Davit is a world-touring saxophonist, composer, producer and creativity coach. His work explores the relationship between our muse – the voice of inspiration, exploration and improvisation – and our editor – the voice of analysis, organization and composition. These two voices play important roles for all creators and serve as counterbalance to the voice of self-doubt and resistance. Steve hopes to inspire other musicians to listen deeply, overcome their obstacles and bring their music into this world. You can discover more about his work at www.SteveDavitMusic.com.

Actually, You Do Have Time for Completing Your Creative Projects

21

Sheila Bender

You are busy! Raising kids, babysitting grandchildren, working, keeping your home running smoothly, caregiving, keeping up communication with family and friends, paying bills, answering email and voicemail. You give yourself time to exercise and shop for healthy food or wait in line for take-out food. If you run your own business or devote time to gardening, volunteering in your community, or helping neighbors with their chores or errands, your ability to find the time to finish your creative projects seems even more diminished, though giving is supposed to inspire love and creativity. You might not even try to get back to your creations and the timeless mindset they require of you – dream time, playing around time, time free of commitments to others.

How are you going to find the time to return to what you have been creating, revisit again and again the joy of working on a project dear to your heart and bring it to fruition?

First, What Is Time?

You've heard time is money. You've heard to use your time wisely. You've heard you must make the most of your time. Ancient Greeks argued about whether time was endless or infinite, linear or cyclical. Scientists and philosophers talk about the time-space continuum. I will leave these discussions to others. And I will leave to others the cliches.

I want to share an analogy about time that will help you find the time you need to finish creative projects. Think of time as windows in a house. When

DOI: 10.4324/9781003351344-21

you are busy, you may open too many windows at once and the creative urge suffers in the strong breeze of to-do items. Other times, you may find there is a window for creativity open a crack, but in desperation, because the opening is so small, you slam the window shut. Sometimes, you believe your window is permanently stuck.

Here are ways to "reframe" time as windows to help you find the time you need to begin and finish your creative projects and start again on new ones.

Are there time-windows you open most often, even regularly, that you don't think of as your creative windows of time – let's call them daily living time-windows – while you don't open creativity time-windows? Instead of refusing to open a creativity window because windows of daily living are open so wide, think of the daily living windows as a bank of windows all on the same side of a room. You don't want lots of air rushing in from the daily living responsibilities with no resistance to help push the air out again. So, from an opposite wall, open at least one creativity window as much as you can, even a crack.

You will soon find the many windows of daily living do not have the "right" to fill the whole room with the stuff of duty. (And isn't creativity the opposite of doing something out of duty, much as you may be invested in doing conscientiously what the due diligence of your life requires?) The fresh breeze of your longing to create will result in a better air balance and you will find you spend more productive time not only on your art but also on your daily administrative duties because your level of boredom and resentment of them will drop considerably.

Okay, but it is one thing to say to do something and that it will work and another to do it.

What to do with whatever air currents you have managed to create? For one, if you can only open the window of your creativity a crack, go with it. You carry around a pen and writing prompts, sketchbook, journal, or pad and spend ten to twenty minutes writing, sketching, working out ideas for where you are going next in your project. I guarantee that you can find the time to create every day – in your car before you go in for an appointment or while the washing machine and dryer are dealing with your clothes or while those you live with are watching television or playing video games. Set an alarm or timer on your device and go to a different room, pretending you have lost the device. Tell yourself that whatever you accomplish in the minutes you allotted to yourself will be worthwhile.

Next time you have the creative window open, it will be easier to get it open wider because doing this work, even if only for ten to twenty minutes, will provide a base you can reread and revisit to reignite the spark you need.

If you do this as much as you can on busy days, when you have a day that allows you to get the window wide open for a longer time, you will have a lot to work with as you begin. The days of these little openings are prep work for keeping the creative wheels greased, wherever you find yourself waiting for someone or able to grab some minutes to create. Otherwise, you may open the creative window wide on a day you do have time for your project and then not have the ability to switch from not creating at all to reentering your project. If that happens, you might find yourself using the wide-open window time for busywork rather than creative work. It takes a lot to overcome the inertia inherent in changing from one state to another. So, by doing the changing in frequent, available small chunks of open windows of limited time, you will get better and better at it. This will help you use the wide-open window of creative time well when you have it.

Maybe there will be a day when you can't get the creativity window open at all. That is when you must envision another window, something like the function of a spare tire (I know this is a mixed metaphor, but mixing it up can free up a creator) and use the time you have for dreaming up a new project and outlining it. Like in a forest where tree roots entwine and help the trees nurture and protect one another, creative roots entwine with current projects and ones just dreamt of. This nurtures both the creator and the ongoing project because the mind is engaged regularly in an oasis of creative ideas rather than the too-often dull ground of everyday responsibilities.

Never accept the idea that time flies and you aren't using yours wisely; if you are in some way working on creativity, you are using time wisely. When you practice this, you will have an easier time moving from the daily state to the flow state of creativity. And thus, you will experience more time.

But what if your creative window really is stuck and not open even a crack and you can't make it budge? How do you open a really stuck window of time? Oh, so many ways! One of my favorites is to read poetry. You are going to find poets who talk your language using observation and evocation, exactly what you thirst to do in your creative work. Some very accessible poets are Billy Collins and Mary Oliver. Others of my go-to poets are David Wagoner, Alison Townsend (who also writes personal essays) and Naomi Shihab Nye, among so many others. There are many poetry organizations with sites online organized to send a poem a day to your inbox.

Another way to unstick the window is to go for a walk and challenge yourself to notice seven things you never noticed before. Sit awhile or return home and write first about what you found yourself thinking or doing instead of purely noticing. Then write about what came alive in you when you did notice. You are unsticking the window by noticing and then by investigating what you had been doing when you weren't noticing – John Keats's term *negative capability* applies here: you are holding one thing and its opposite in the same work. Life is full of one thing and its opposite and we use the fraternal twins in our creations, but we can also make ourselves see them in our daily lives. Then the window opens. You are creating. You will feel refreshed, not stale and can take up your projects to see what negative capability they include: as, in this case, when you noticed what noticing was like and what not noticing was like.

Life is full and you can use that fullness to provide the substrate of your work, if only you use whatever windows of time you have to do your work and bring it to fruition only to start again creating more. That is what creators do. Learning to enjoy the practice in small steps, you will celebrate the large accomplishments of finishing and eagerly get back to the small steps for creating something new.

Three Tips for Creatives

1. Write three sentences about time that keep you judging the creating time you have as inadequate. Cross them out. Crumple the paper you wrote them on and toss those sentences to the wind or into the garbage can.
2. Write three more sentences about your creating time-window with specific ways you will open it. Keep those sentences in your purse or pocket or on your car dashboard or dresser top.
3. Open your creating window every day by using whatever time you can find to generate ideas or work on some aspect of your project, even if it is a very small amount of work. The inertia that keeps you from opening the creating window is overcome by inch-by-inch openings.

Three Tips for Coaches

1. Ask clients to make a list of three things that keep them from finishing a creative project and practice turning their words into action items. For example, "I don't want to get started because I'll be interrupted" can become "Interruptions often bring new

inspiration. It is okay to work and have to stop for a while because of an interruption."

2. Ask clients to visualize a "creating window" inside a structure that they don't usually think of as a place to create. For instance, if they are in their car, then before going into the store or while waiting for someone, they might make a list of the steps needed to finish a project and put those steps in their calendar instead of spending those few minutes checking email or visiting social media.

3. Have the client write a journal entry about their creative window, when they've opened it and what they've accomplished while it was open.

 ## About the Author

Sheila Bender is the founder of WritingItReal.com, a website for those who write from personal experience. She teaches writers' workshops online and in person. Her books on writing include *A Year in the Life: Journaling for Self-Discovery* and *Writing Personal Poetry: Creating Poems from Your Personal Experiences*, both available through the International Association for Journal Writing. Her memoir, *A New Theology: Turning to Poetry in a Time of Grief* and *Since Then: Poems and Short Prose* are her newest works.

Finding a Kinder Way to Let Go **22**

Ahava Shira

It was a cold evening in late December 2009. I was on the verge of finishing my doctoral dissertation in language and literacy education, after two years of researching, writing and editing the 200-page manuscript, a manuscript composed of equal parts narrative, poetry, photography and the requisite theoretical text and scholarly citations.

Sitting in my favorite white chair beside the woodstove, light fading from the skylight above, I dialed the phone number of my professor and academic supervisor, Dr. Carl Leggo.

"I liked it how it was previously, Carl; it was beautiful and I like it now," I admitted, having spent the entire day rearranging various quotations in the thesis.

I can hear Dr. Leggo's words now, just as he said them then, in his warm laugh of a voice, full of wisdom from years of his own laboring with words. A poet and proud parent of my PhD, he replied, "I think it is time to let go, Ahava."

I have come to recognize how the phases of a creative project are like the phases of the moon. Although the new, waxing and full phases all have their thrills and challenges, it is the waning phase of the cycle that I want to explore here. Better yet, let's call it *weaning*. Because, like it or not, it's what we all have to do to bring the project we have been working on to completion.

Let's start with a definition, adapted from a few different web sources:

> Wean: cause to quit something or let go of that which one has desired, striven for, depended on, been addicted to, been accustomed to, or been habituated to.

DOI: 10.4324/9781003351344-22

Depending on its size, scale and scope and our relationship with it, our creative project may become a habit, a devotion, an obsession and/ or an addiction. Like an infant needing us to help them become the adult they are meant to be, every creative project requires focus, continued attention, concentration and care. We become attached to it, out of joyful connection and impassioned responsibility. This means that when the time comes, we must find our way through the process of detaching, or weaning. Again, depending on the project, this will require different skills, timing and action.

I have not always had an easy time with weaning myself from my creative projects. I much prefer being in the midst of the creative flowing than the letting go. First drafts are my joy. I also value the continuation, the ongoing inquiry and reflection, the editing and playing around with form.

Perhaps the challenge is that I keep expecting the letting go to be easy, or easier. Whether it was my first poetry book, my first memoir, or the one I am currently writing, completing each of these projects has taken far more time, energy, focus and commitment than anticipated.

Is that because I am a bad planner? Do I have unrealistic expectations? Do I work slowly? Perhaps it's because every creative project stretches me in new ways. Moreover, there is always the wondering about the is-there-more-that-I-can-do-to-improve-it? question.

Despite this, I have finished so many creative projects in my 55 years that I can now honestly say I do know how to let go. Meaning I have learned how to wean myself. More precisely, I have learned that there are many ways to lean into, as opposed to avoiding, the weaning. You are probably already in the midst of one or some of them:

- Accepting a deadline, whether self-imposed or other expected
- Moving to addressing the next stage of a project, like editorial support, publication, or performance
- Responding to an opportunity or the desire to share the work
- Recognizing that you have read the manuscript many times and keep making the same changes over and over again
- Inviting another to support and escort you into it

In the conversation with my professor, all these figured in. What I have learned is that when it comes to creative projects, weaning is inevitable and necessary. Still, we may find ourselves resisting and turning away. However, if we do choose to stay the course toward completion, it helps not to criticize or condemn ourselves if we are finding it difficult. Kindness and compassion are much better, softer, easier ways to help us let go.

It's also good to remember that, in the case of creative projects:

- There is no such thing as perfection.
- We will always think it can be better.
- We will doubt the quality of the work.
- We won't be sure it's good enough.
- We will ask ourselves, "But what if I just did that or that or that?"
- A B+ is better than an unfinished project, as my husband has taken to saying recently.

If you are having a challenging time of it, here are a few writing prompts to go to the page with:

- How might I practice kindness toward myself in this process of weaning?
- Why would I not want to let go? Why would I want to let go?
- What would make this letting go more easeful, more peaceful?
- Who can I ask for support in this process?

 Three Tips for Creatives

1. Rather than "begin with the end in mind," as Stephen Covey, author of *7 Habits of Highly Effective People* suggests, end with the beginning (of your next project) in mind and let yourself be carried over the completion threshold by the unknown poetry within your next process of artistic creation.
2. Practice *kindf*ulness all the way through your weaning process.
3. Allow yourself to receive the help of those who have found peaceful, easeful ways of letting go.

 Three Tips for Coaches

1. Remember how it felt the first time you had to wean yourself from a creative project. Remember the fear, the anger, the frustration. Feel compassion for yourself and bring that into your exchange with your clients.

2. Even coaches and mentors have a hard time letting go. Go easy the next time you have to meet a deadline for a new course or group program. What can you do to wean yourself gently?
3. Study the moon. Learn to recognize its cycles. This will help you know where you are and where your clients are.

 ## About the Author

Dr. Ahava Shira (she/her) is a poet, dancer, filmmaker, memoir writer, mentor and facilitator, living on the unceded traditional territory of the Coast Salish Peoples (Salt Spring Island, BC). Dedicated to creating safe and ethical spaces for personal nourishment and collective transformation, Ahava helps creatives develop strategies for coping with the impacts of inner and outer change through expressing difficult emotions, cultivating joy and compassion and shaping a new story for their relationship with themselves, with all beings and with the earth. Her current pleasures include beach dancing, forest walking and falling in love again and again with her beloved husband and this beautiful planet earth.

A Creative Structure for Completion

23

Cindy Yantis

Completion takes guts. It also takes verve, time, sweat, planning and maybe a couple of Tylenol when a deadline is looming.

It takes strategy and structure.

The idea of structure is often left brain and for a creative, it can feel rigid, the antithesis of creation. But when you bring your creativity as strategy, it can become a game. And, if you dive into it with play and curiosity, structure is not only effective but can be fun.

Creating structure for completing your important work is vital. As in creating an outline for a book, a work structure provides the framework to contain your efforts.

When a Structure is Finite, You Can be Infinite Within It

As creatives and coaches for creatives, we often deal with being scattered. We know what it's like to fall in love with and get distracted by ideas and shiny objects. The start-and-stop way of being keeps us from fulfilling our promise and purpose. It keeps us from completion.

Research shows that interruptions derail your attention. It can take up to twenty-five minutes to, once again, reach deep focus. We all know the rabbit hole awaiting us if we open or heed the interrupting notification. Following a link can culminate in hours of wasted time and overworked brain cells. And unfinished work. Pretty soon, we're completely off task rather than completing the task at hand.

DOI: 10.4324/9781003351344-23

Which is why a commitment to a finite structure is key for completing your important work.

The following is a structure method I've used and have shared with clients.

The 28-Minute Time Capsule

What does it mean to be infinite in a finite structure? It means being free within a prearranged set of parameters designed to aid productivity and creativity so you don't pay attention to anything but the creative project in front of you.

It was inspiration and desperation that caused me to first tap into this time capsule method. I was under deadline and feeling overwhelmed with a scattered to-do list. I decided to set a timer to stay on task.

"Twenty-eight minutes" popped into my head, so I set the timer for twenty-eight minutes. My attention wandered at around six minutes, but because of the timer, I refocused. Before I knew it, the twenty-eight minutes was up and I was in flow. I pressed repeat and finished the project before deadline. It only took about three twenty-eight-minute time capsules because I was in deep focus on that one project only.

Setting a timer was not revolutionary, but it felt that way to me. In fact, it was a game changer, so I started sharing it with clients and associates.

My client – I'll call her Lou – was a busy teacher and astrologer. She had a hard time staying committed to her weekly newsletter.

After distilling her confronting issues, it came down to a feeling of overload. Lou had so many messages she wanted to convey to her readers that they stopped the spigot. I suggested we brainstorm a list of topics and use the time capsule method for each topic.

She knew once she was able to focus on one message and carve out time to write, it wouldn't take her long to complete. She was able to front-load several months' worth of newsletters. It diminished her sense of overload.

The Power of 28

After some success with the time capsule, I started wondering about the number 28. I learned the number 28 connects to nature, space, science and math. It also aligns with ancient wisdom that correlates to the universal clock into which we are all tuned.

Some Fun Tidbits About the Number 28

- In math, 28 is a perfect number. There are only four perfect numbers identified in ancient times: 6; 28; 496; and 8,128.
- In numerology, 28 signifies a beginning and an end: $2 + 8 = 10$ and $1 + 0 = 1$. One is the alpha (beginning). Ten is the omega (end).
- There are 28 days in a solar moon cycle.
- There are 28 days in a woman's menstrual cycle.
- Buddha contemplated for 28 days under the fig tree.
- There are 28 letters in the Danish, Swedish, Arabic and Esperanto alphabets.
- A human being has 28 teeth (minus the wisdom teeth).
- It takes 28 heartbeats for a red globule to circuit the entire body.
- There are 28 dominos in a box of dominos.
- There are 28 petals in a perfect rose.
- The melting point of butter starts at 28 degrees C.
- It takes 28 days for the surface of the sun to fully rotate.
- It takes Saturn approximately 28 years to revolve around the sun.

Could the number 28 be sacred? Is the number 28 integral in the creation of time? Could that mean that the number 28 taps you into your universal time clock?

Who knows? But I do know the twenty minute time capsule works in helping you to intend, focus and complete.

One client – I'll call her Liz – felt overwhelmed facing a massive project. Not a writer, she was asked to contribute a chapter to a book. The approaching deadline crippled her as fear sabotaged her focus.

Asking her why she was invited to be a book contributor reminded her of her expertise. It diminished the fear. We divided the project into bite-size chunks. I suggested the time capsule, concentrating on one topic per capsule.

The upshot was, she had a solid structure and was able to build momentum once she started to see progress. Capsule by capsule.

Building Your Time Capsule

The historical purpose of a time capsule is to capture life at a moment in time. A well-built time capsule is seamless and sealed to secure and protect the space.

It's a useful metaphor to create your twenty minute time capsule for completion.

Start with a question: "What will support me to focus and be my most prolific?"

Here are key things to consider for succeeding in your time capsule:

- Environment. The best environment involves seating, lighting, privacy and sound to get comfortable and set the right energy and tone for optimal creativity. For sound, silence or instrumental music is best.
- Tools. Gather writing utensils, paintbrushes, notebook, laptop/tablet, recording device and noise-cancelling headphones.
- Body hydration and satiation. Keep hydrated. Make sure you're not hungry or too full. High-protein, healthy foods support brain function and focus.
- Timer. Best to use a portable timer. If you use your phone, turn off notifications and select a non-jarring alarm so as not to interrupt flow, like chimes or bells.
- Clear the space. Close all windows and distractions. Try using only one monitor.
- Time of day. Choose the time when you're typically most productive and creative. You can follow your circadian rhythm. Are you a morning lark or a night owl?
- Intention. Once you identify the topic, set the intention to focus and complete.
- Pre-capsule prep. Take two to five minutes to breathe deeply and center yourself.
- Track. Treat each completed capsule as a milestone to celebrate on your path to completion. It builds momentum.

A group time capsule can be effective, in person or online.

One client, a screenwriter, sets up an early morning "writer's room" on Zoom for fellow writers to join him. Everyone joins in and states their intentions in the chat for that session. He provides the time capsule.

Each writer sets their timer. Together, they're committed to the sacred and intentional space of the Zoom room.

After three consecutive time capsule sessions, it's a good idea to take a short fifteen minute break. Stretch. Hydrate. Close your eyes. Reassess.

Then enter the time capsule and begin again.

Twenty minute time capsule template:

Identify. Focus. Complete. Repeat. Track.

- *Identify* one project to complete.
- *Focus* fully.
- *Complete* the twenty-eight minutes – then assess.
- *Repeat* twenty-eight minutes on this project or move on to another.
- *Track* your milestones toward completion.

Identify. Focus. Complete. Repeat. Track.

To-Do List versus Time Capsule List

A to-do list is broad. A time capsule list is specific. Take one item from the to-do list and capsule it into completable and progressive chunks.

Estimate how many 28-minute time capsules it will take to complete the full project. Schedule them into your calendar.

There are 1,440 minutes in 24 hours and 480 minutes in each 8-hour day. And seventeen 28-minute time capsule opportunities within those 8 hours.

For this chapter, I estimated the following on my time capsule list:

- 1–2 capsules for client stories
- 1–2 capsules for research
- 5 capsules for the rough draft
- 3 capsules for the edit and polish

Once you do a few, you have a good grasp on how long it will take and it becomes easier to meet or beat your deadlines.

 Three Tips for Creatives

1. Break your project into manageable, completable, trackable chunks.
2. Be curious and playful as you create your time capsule for optimal creation.
3. Celebrate each milestone on your progress to completion.

Three Tips for Coaches

1. Help guide your client to unpack and break down a large or looming project.
2. Ask probing questions to glean exactly what's stopping them from completing. Finding the time and space are often obstacles. Introduce this creative way to structure their project into time capsule sessions. It can be a game changer.
3. Help them track and celebrate their momentum and progress. When you're committed to the time capsule, you don't have to worry about managing your attention. When you're committed to the time capsule, it's easier to concentrate and focus. Research shows that the brain changes when you focus for longer periods more often. The brain rewires its neuroplasticity and neural networks. Over time, this strategy for completing creative work gets easier.

    The twenty minute time capsule is great for other things too: administrative duties, email, social media, or housework. You'll be amazed at what you can accomplish and complete in a day.

 About the Author

Cindy Yantis is a writer and creativity coach with vast experience in creative writing, screenwriting, advertising and business. She helps clients get to the heart of their stories. She understands the struggle with creative process and the fears that stand in the way of true creative potential. Through trial and error, she knows what works and what doesn't. Find out more at www.cin dyyantis.com.

The Quest(ions) to Completion

24

Lessons in Following Your Bliss

Erin Hallagan Clare

In the summer of 2015, I made the decision I was going to at long last start my own business: an arts space dedicated to storytelling through all art mediums. The plan was to finish out the year at my job, find a property and then jump in headfirst.

I suddenly had the energy of two people. While tending to my already-demanding career, I somehow found time to form an LLC, build a website, write a business plan and learn QuickBooks. (Okay, the last one's a lie, but I tried.) Summer turned into fall, fall into winter and at the moment of no return . . . I chickened out.

At dinner with my boss, as I fumbled through an attempt to give notice, she presented a counteroffer: a salary increase *and* the opportunity to take dedicated time in our off-season to work on the business.

I accepted. But despite this gift of time, I completely lost all momentum. Before I even started, I felt like a failure, simply because things weren't going precisely according to plan.

Weeks of paralysis went by. Eventually, I began to differentiate between the messages hailing from my ego and my soul and asked, "Who am I going to let run the show?"

In response, I decided to inch my way forward and focus on building a foundation, brick by brick. This shift in perspective was groundbreaking. Rather than opening a physical venue right out of the gate, I began programming pop-up arts events at all sorts of different spaces. Slowly but surely, people started showing up.

DOI: 10.4324/9781003351344-24

And along the way, I learned what it took to outfit an outdoor venue versus a banquet hall versus an intimate listening room. I learned what type of equipment was necessary and trusted the voice deep down telling me to record every event. I learned how to communicate with our patrons. (*Parking! Always share how to find parking!*) I learned stage presence and how not to be terrified of the microphone. I discovered more people read our newsletter on Tuesdays at 2:00 p.m. than on Thursdays at 4:00 p.m., with the bulk of their responses being "How do I learn how to tell my own story? I'd love to participate someday."

So I learned how to teach. I watched the video archive of folks sharing their work and saw *story* at the core of it all. I asked, "How does one excavate their personal narrative and repurpose it for creative bounty?" Soon, classes and workshops were added into the fold.

All of a sudden, it was 2017 and I realized months had gone by when I hadn't even thought about a venue. I started visiting properties. There was this one place – a former dance studio – where I could truly visualize the space. The stage could go in the corner and if the south-facing wall was opened up, there would be plenty of room for seating. And the storage area in back? A classroom, easily. Plus, the money made from three years of events and workshops would cover start-up costs.

After some back-and-forth lease negotiations and everything looking promising, the owner called to say they had decided to sell the lot to a convenience store instead. This happened, in various iterations, numerous times thereafter.

As 2018 rolled along, I found out I was pregnant. My son arrived in December and once again, the notion of a physical space was put back on the shelf.

In the hours between nursing and easing into my new role as a mother, I revisited what drew me to this concept in the first place and remembered one of my favorite quotes by Joseph Campbell: "If you follow your bliss, you put yourself on a kind of track that has been there all the while, waiting for you and the life that you ought to be living is the one you are living."

And so, although it wasn't linear or part of the original road map, I enrolled in a creativity coaching program. I studied the art and psychology of creativity and put them into practice within my own work. I saw the staggering parallels between starting an arts business and starting an art project. And while I had yet to fully realize my vision, in my bones, I still felt I was on the right path, so I created a mantra, B.L.I.S.S., to help navigate my way to the finish line. I trust it can help you get to the finish line of your creative pursuits as well.

B.L.I.S.S.

Begin and begin again. With each setback, begin again and with a beginner's mind, consider where you can loosen the grip on your original vision and let the creative process inform its evolution more effortlessly toward the end. How can you infuse the energy and excitement of the beginning into each next step?

Learn and unlearn. Creativity offers some of the greatest invitations for personal growth. It has the power to swiftly reveal our shadows and struggles. By working through these lessons in our creative endeavors, we are simultaneously supporting our ongoing development as human beings. We are unlearning old ways of being, strengthening our proverbial muscles and proving to ourselves we are capable of traversing the spectrum from concept to completion. Creativity and knowledge aren't fixed commodities. How can you engage a growth mindset?

Inquire within. Ask questions – lots of them! – and let your subconscious go to work (one of the most powerful tools in a creative practice). Bring a sense of inquiry to the meaning that would arise not only from finishing a project but also within yourself as an artist. Pursue intuitive clues rather than fixating on the way things are "supposed" to be. Where can you live with the questions as opposed to assuming the answers?

Small steps. Often the biggest barrier to completing creative work is focusing on the final product and not the process needed to get there. Break things down and then break them down smaller. This ultimately fosters new habits, impacts long-lasting change and moves us through resistance. When in doubt, my all-time favorite question is from my teacher, Eric Maisel: what is the next right thing?

Show up. Build the habit, the practice and the perspectives that serve and the courage to create. The trick is to keep moving. Momentum begets momentum, creativity begets creativity and the best remedy to feeling stuck is to take action. Oh and don't forget to play! What is something you can do to enjoy the journey of creating just a little bit more?

When COVID Hit

When COVID hit, my husband and I made the decision to move closer to family. We found a darling house in the mountains of Asheville, North Carolina and read up on what to do in the event of any bear encounters. I at last quit my job and spent my days working with students and clients in navigating their own unique creative quests.

As for my dream of an arts venue, I kept my feather duster handy and let it know I'd be back when the time was right.

Sure enough, in the fall of 2021, I stumbled upon a vacant brick building (circa the 1920s) while on a walk in West Asheville. It had floor to ceiling arched storefront windows, a loft space, hardwood floors, tin ceilings and a magical energy about it. I called our realtor, scheduled a tour and, within three months, was handed the keys to what from that day forth would be called Story Parlor. And while it has the roots and seeds of its predecessor, its blossoms are entirely its own.

 Three Tips for Creatives

1. Where can you lower the pressure and add more compassion for the feelings of fear and resistance that will inevitably ebb and flow? This is a practice of accepting the natural response to navigating the unknown (i.e., creativity!), as well as getting past barriers such as perfectionism, procrastination, doubt and a harsh inner critic.

2. How can you reframe the idea of success in a way that allows you to actually be successful? Our brains value success experiences, so, literally set yourself up for it, perhaps building in designated pit stops en route to the finish line. Each "win" chisels away at unhelpful, engrained narratives that are often responsible for our creative blocks. Be sure to celebrate those successes along the way!

3. When feeling stuck, what is in your power to change and what is out of your hands? With the latter, is there any room to change your perspective? (As Erich Heller said, "Be careful how you interpret the world: it is that way.") Regarding what *is* in your control, ask yourself this: of all the things you could possibly do to move this project along and impact positive change, which one will you choose to do?

Three Tips for Coaches

1. Normalize the hard parts of the process. Remind clients that creativity and difficulty are synonymous (they bring us to our knees *and* lift us up), encouraging them to let go of dualistic ways of thinking. Finding a way to accept that the journey will be both hard *and* rewarding – not just one or the other – clears the path toward completion and, in turn, cultivates a more resilient creative spirit. Invite them to ponder, "What could make the next small step a little easier?"
2. Empower a sense of autonomy. Move the client from a place of victimization ("I can't do this"; "I don't know how to do this"; "This is too hard for me") to mastery ("I perhaps don't know how to do this right now, but I trust that I can figure it out"). Ask them about the times they've completed similar things in the past and what worked for them – or what they think *could* work now – bringing them into their own sense of power and capability.
3. Provide opportunities to check in regarding meaning. Ask thought-provoking, investigative questions such as, "What are you passionate about within this piece?" "What questions do you want to explore about yourself and your worldview in this process?" "What would it mean to you and about you, to complete this project?" This is the necessary fuel to meet the fulfillment both of self and of project.

About the Author

Erin Hallagan Clare is the founder and artistic director of Story Parlor, a cooperative arts venue in Asheville, North Carolina, dedicated to storytelling and the exploration of the human condition through community-driven programming. She is a certified creativity coach and Enneagram practitioner and is completing her Master's in Psychology with a creativity studies specialization. A writer and a storyteller, her work has been featured in *Psychology Today, Thrive Global, Austin Monthly* and others. More information can be found at www.storyparloravl.com or www.inwardandartward.com.

How Pietro Used Discipline and Self-imposed Constraints to Complete His Artistic Project

25

Coleen Chandler

In business, the success of a project depends on keenly managing constraints such as costs, schedules, scope, benefits, time and quality. Alter one piece of this puzzle – less money or time, for example – and quality will suffer; so goes the conventional wisdom. Therefore, the job of a project manager is to smooth out, reckon with and manage constraints, so as to deliver the best product possible.

Many creatives believe that they must eliminate all constraints to allow for maximum flexibility and inspiration in the creative process in order to produce their best work. Pietro, an illustrator and a client, was firmly in that camp. The mere idea of constraints made him suffocate and brought forth the rebel in him. But what if his broad freedom had started to work against him and hindered his ability to complete his artistic projects?

So, what exactly is a constraint? A constraint is a limiting factor put on a project or action. Think of Twitter. One must focus and deliver a clear point of view in a certain limited number of characters. What about tiny homes? I marvel at the ingenuity of architects who can use every ounce of their creativity to design livable homes in a 225-square-foot floor plan. And finally, for the sports fans among us, what would sports be without lines, goalposts and timers?

DOI: 10.4324/9781003351344-25

In each of these examples, the excitement comes from the challenge of writing, creating and playing within the well-defined boundaries we accept. To fully excel, we do our best to shine within these constraints with determination and discipline.

Constraints can be outwardly imposed, such as a publisher's deadline, or self-imposed. The rest of the chapter focuses on self-imposed constraints and how they helped Pietro submit his project on time. The question we posed was how the use of constraints might help him enhance his creative process and complete his artistic project. That's the challenge we took on.

Pietro was hired by a major publisher to produce twelve illustrations for a children's book. This was his big break and the pressure was on. When he came to me for support, he had completed seven illustrations during a four-month period and the remaining five were due in six weeks. This was a firm deadline. He was panicking and felt he had taken on a project out of his league, which created an ominous sense of failure and inadequacy.

His mind was racing.

Pietro: Why did I accept this project? It's obvious I'm not up to the task. I run around in circles in my studio like a caged animal. I can't focus, my thoughts are all over the place, I feel I'm imploding, my sketches suck and now I'm running out of time. I'm stressed to the max. What's going to happen if I don't deliver?

Coach: It does sound stressful, Pietro. You say you run around in circles in your studio. Can you describe your studio?

Pietro: It's gorgeous. It's upstairs, a large room with windows all around overlooking a lush yard and, in the distance, a mountain range. I'm so blessed and can dream for hours here watching the changing scenery. It's my favorite room in the house. Right now, however, I'm not feeling productive.

Coach: One week ago, we introduced the concept of time constraints and working within strict scheduling guidelines to help you focus better. That didn't appeal to you at first. However, you said today that you're starting to see some benefits. Would you be willing to try environmental constraints as well?

Pietro: Like what?

Coach: Well, I'll let you tell me. You seem to be spending a lot of energy running around your studio, possibly distracted by its gorgeous views as well. Would that energy better serve you if it were more focused, contained within a smaller space, perhaps? What would that look like?

Pietro: No way. I need space, breathing room, lots of space, or I feel trapped.

Coach: How is that "lots of space" working for you right now?

Pietro: It's not.

Coach: Ah, so . . .

Pietro: Okay, I see what you mean. I've nothing to lose after all. Let me come up with something.

After some back and forth, with Pietro at once laughing and panicking as his workspace shrank with each iteration, he decided to go all in and use his bedroom walk-in closet. It had good light, thanks to a skylight and enough room for a small table, easel and stool.

We did a visualization exercise to help him center himself and deal with the claustrophobic sensation of a closed-in space. He envisioned himself relaxed, excited and creative in that small space and came up with a couple of rituals to help him enter and settle himself in the closet. We even added a dash of humor around boogeymen for good measure.

A week passed.

Coach: How did it go, Pietro?

Pietro: You won't believe it. The first three days, I was miserable. Spending eight to ten hours a day in that closet was rough. I fought it, but I admit that I sensed that the smaller space was becoming beneficial. Then I remembered our discussion on time constraints and how precise I needed to be. So, instead of an open day flowing at will, I decided to give myself defined chunks of time throughout the day, two hours at a time with exactly twenty-minute breaks in between, plus an hour for lunch and one hour for dinner. And, do you know what? It worked. I finished an illustration in four days. My absolute record.

Coach: Wow, that's impressive. What a shift! You sound so excited. What happened to the trapped animal?

Pietro: Desperation, Coleen. I had no choice. I relaxed and told it to take a hike, just like we talked about. Three weeks ago, it would have been unimaginable to me that I could work out of such a confined space and actually be creative and productive.

Coach: And now?

Pietro: I have four illustrations to do in four weeks. It's insane when you think about it, but I've proven to myself I can do it. I believe I can do it! I can't wait to get back to my studio. What a reward that will be for me, but in the meantime, it's TTC [tiny creative closet] all the way.

By creating his own self-imposed time and environmental constraints, Pietro was able to reduce distractions and deliver his illustrations on time. He also demonstrated a crucial quality to make this process possible: discipline. Without discipline, he would have been unable to stick to his grueling schedule.

Discipline is the twin sibling of constraint. Self-imposed constraints do not work if one lacks the discipline to stick to them. Together, they multiply the artist's ability to be productive and creative.

Pietro was both amazed at the results brought on by this new discipline of constraints and relieved that he could go back to his beloved studio. True to his promise to himself, he had set foot in it only to get supplies for his art.

Pietro observed:

> I've learned so much through this process. I busted through ingrained ideas on the creative process that have held me back. I was able to get over my fear of small spaces and turn that into an asset. I noticed my reluctance to be disciplined at first, then I went all in by surrendering to it. I feel pride at having kept my word to myself. And I'm humbled that I created some of my best work in a clothes closet, when I have a beautiful studio at my disposal. Constraints and TTC are in my future – for real.

Three Tips for Creatives

1. Never forget: it's your choice. Embracing the discipline of constraints is an exploration into the unknown, a challenge and a proven path to completion. Trust yourself.
2. Be creative with constraints. Invent your own, study how your favorite artists use them, try a few and give yourself the chance to fully experience them. Don't give up too quickly. The gift of completion is on the other side.
3. Let go of your preconceived notions on creativity, freedom, discipline and constraints. Broaden your meaning of these words. How else can you think about them to help you complete your creative project?

Three Tips for Coaches

1. Encourage your creative clients to try constraints. The operative word is **try**. Nothing permanent, nothing scary, just a try. Creatives as a whole balk at the idea of being boxed in. Give them breathing

room to explore and reframe constraints to fit their needs and let them come up with their own.

2. Turn discipline into a joyous process in which the artist's sense of freedom and agency lie in determining their own self-imposed limits and staying true to their word.

3. Stay firm. Don't buy into your client's fear story that they can't do it. Completing a project is hard for any creative, so keep being the strong voice that holds them through that journey by being an unconditional ambassador for the power of constraints and discipline.

 ## About the Author

Coleen Chandler, ICF-PCC, CPCC, is an accomplished creativity and performance coach who works with artists, performers and creative entrepreneurs to help them strategize, focus and execute their creative visions – often difficult undertakings for creatives to achieve on their own. A performing songwriter herself, she specializes in the performing arts, conquering stage fright and speaking with confidence. Her moto: let's get it done! Coleen is a Professional Certified Coach (PCC) through the International Coaching Federation (ICF) and a mentor coach. She serves on the board of the ICF Sacramento Chapter as Director of Credentialing. You can reach her at coleen@coleen chandler.com.

Working From the Inside Out

26

Jackie Beaver

Completion is not always about finishing a piece or ending a task. Sometimes it's about reaching a point that feels right in order to move on in our work – a kind of resetting. Just as we declutter and reorganize space, sometimes we embark on an internal working out of needs, desires and priorities. As coaching is often seen as dynamic and focused support to help get things done, I got to wondering about a curious meandering experience I had with a client I'll call Mary.

She called me about doing some creativity coaching. Her voice had a certain energy; her words spilled over in a flood of information about herself and her work. I felt slightly overwhelmed, especially when she made it clear that she was definitely not looking for creative stimulation but help in gaining "recognition." Could I help?

Mary was retired and had practiced her art alongside a day job. She had grown up in the countryside and left when she was quite young to settle in a city where she still lived. She hadn't had much contact with her family for some years. She told me that she felt they had never really understood her. She said she was thinking a lot about where she had come from and what she might do next. She seemed to be a woman with strong convictions, both active and engaged. She had forged her own artistic path and had a cultural network.

She worked with "materials" but declared that she was neither craftsperson nor artisan. She was an artist because she was motivated by convictions and a need to express herself creatively. She added wistfully that she was no good at "selling" and that she didn't exhibit her work in traditional art galleries. Mary expressed a feeling of not belonging in mainstream art circles

DOI: 10.4324/9781003351344-26

because she was "self-taught." She wanted to be recognized for her art and yet wondered whether it was legitimate to desire recognition at her age. She was sixty-seven years old at the time.

I was touched by this. We live in a world where youth, beauty and energy prevail. How do aging creatives find their place in it, especially those who, having retired from a day job, can finally give more time to their creative work?

I wondered how artists could gain recognition without exhibitions or sales. I felt that we needed to investigate this thing, "recognition." What did it mean to Mary? What did it look like? She agreed. Yes, that was the point! She wasn't sure herself and needed help structuring her thoughts about how she could show who and what she was. She said she'd reached a stage in life where she needed to assemble and reassemble the threads of her creative work. I asked Mary to jot down some thoughts about "recognition."

We agreed to talk over the course of the following three months. No money was exchanged. I knew that I couldn't guarantee she'd find "recognition," but I could perhaps help her unravel her thoughts. Each week seemed to bring something new: a current preoccupation, a memory, an account of what she had done in the past week. Diligent efforts to keep us focused on "recognition" were often frustrated. I realized later that this was why she had come to me. *Help me get a clearer picture of what I want. I am full of thoughts and ideas; help me sort them out.*

The need for organization extended to actual things too. She had lost her studio space, so materials and tools encumbered her and her husband's living space. There was an urgent need to address this.

Mary identified that sharing and communicating were important elements of "recognition" for her. She was involved in several collaborative projects at the time. She talked about them a lot. Mary said she felt that her work was seen and valued by other artists. She said that she was beginning to look at these experiences differently. She was noticing that both she and her work were received and perceived within the context of forming a new "work." She said that she was growing more aware that collaboration gave her opportunities to transmit her ideas, her experience and her know-how to younger artists. She felt valued, energized, recognized.

One day, Mary announced that she was applying for a city arts grant to help her establish a new studio. This seemed a positive step toward action. I asked how she thought a grant might help. What would she use the money for? She mentioned storage solutions, even maybe a separate room to store her materials. I wondered at the likelihood of receiving funding for that. However, I wanted to be encouraging and suggested she start putting together her application. The process would be useful as she had mentioned wanting to review, reorganize and update her portfolio.

The following week, Mary was at a dead end. She said she couldn't propose a budget or a time scale for a specific aspect of a project, apart from identifying some cupboards she needed and she realized that these didn't have a direct bearing on her latest artistic research. However, she was absorbed in digging through old files and rediscovering projects from way back. She was revisiting past work and considering how some of it could be useful now. Mary reflected that "recognition" could also come from within, through retrospection, taking stock of one's artistic journey and accepting one's own creative work like accepting oneself.

Mary also talked about a contact she'd made with a new arts coworking association. Did she want to set up on her own or with a larger group? I was perplexed. Should I help her decide which way to go or leave her to find her own way? Only Mary could know what was right for her. All I could do was listen, reflect back and ask questions as she worked it out.

I asked regularly about the grant application and the arts cooperative, but there wasn't much to tell. Mary was keener on talking about her work, past and present. She reported that she was continuing to jot down thoughts about herself, exploring her artistic identity and developing ideas about her place as an aging artist.

Mary seemed to be using our sessions to sift through her past, share about the present and wonder about her future. One time, she said, "I don't want to give all my energy away." She was talking about the effort of establishing links and working with others or setting up a studio on her own. She knew that effort was required, but she did not want to deplete herself. Even though I understood her concern, I was also frustrated by a sense of inertia and felt we were going nowhere.

As we neared the end of three months, Mary announced that she was going on holiday and was also visiting her family, saying she had decided to reopen that part of her life. Just before leaving, she was meeting up with the arts cooperative as well. This was like fresh air to me. I was glad Mary would have a change of scenery. Her upcoming meeting with the cooperative was also positive, even though she was apprehensive. Would she like them, would they like her, would their ethos align with hers? I was glad to have a break myself.

When Mary returned, she was in a whirlwind of excitement. Her holiday had been great and she had renewed ties with her family. She had also joined the arts cooperative and was moving into shared studio space. The group was preparing a launch event and she had already been interviewed to promote it. Mary reflected that this was what she had been looking for – to be accepted and be part of a group of working artists in which each member was valued for their creative input, recognized by the others and recognized as a group by the public.

Mary had found some recognition, some validation and a feeling of having a place in the cultural landscape and a space in which to practice. But had our sessions actually helped? I had mostly listened and asked questions. Mary had pulled me along on her own meandering journey.

Not so long ago, she messaged me, saying that she'd been thinking about how our sessions had helped her realize what she was looking for and recognize the opportunities for finding it. Mary reminded me that listening to someone with interest, providing appropriate encouragement and giving them space to ventilate thoughts and ideas so they could sift through and reorganize them were basic yet fundamental coaching tools. These tools can help clients reset on the inside in order for them to move on in their work with renewed energy and confidence.

Three Tips for Creatives

1. Try to put a name to what you are searching for or hoping for in your creative work. Then explore what it really means for you. Give it more definition. This can help orient your reflections and investigations.
2. Review creative work with a critical but kind eye. How do you feel about it now? How did it come to be made? What themes emerge? Write down your thoughts and reflections. They could help you learn more about your creative needs and desires and, as a result, help you in formulating your next steps.
3. It can be helpful to have someone to talk to openly and without judgment who can give you some time, actively listen and help you keep on track.

Three Tips for Coaches

1. Listen, listen, listen and reflect back. We can forget to listen and get caught up identifying problems and finding solutions. Being listened to and feeling understood can help clients feel validated in their work and in their person and, consequently, more confident about finding their own solutions.
2. Providing a framework for clients to wander through their thoughts is similar to giving them an exercise to experience making a mess. Work on creating this framework.
3. Within the structure of a coaching session, clients are free to talk about whatever they need to while coaches can provide an anchor by asking questions and reminding clients of their initial objectives.

About the Author

Jackie Beaver is an art therapist and creativity coach based in Switzerland. She works with children and adults. She has a background in education and is interested in experiential learning.

Finishing Paintings   **27**

Anni Barsoum

I started painting in 1987 after the birth of my daughter. As soon as the babies had gone to bed, I would run to my easel in the dining room and spend hours painting still life paintings and landscapes with oils. Two mornings a week, I took art classes at the Dubai Art Center. A year later, the third baby came into our lives. Soon after the delivery, I returned to work in a bank. I put away the canvases and brushes. My recently started artistic career was put on hold.

Thirty years later, in the fall of 2017, with all three children in new nests and pondering my next steps in the journey of life, I found myself applying for a Color of Woman certification. In those pre-COVID days, living in Abu Dhabi on the flight path between the Americas and Australia and used to a life of travel, I was as attracted to the in-person workshops in different locations as I was to learning the 13-step process.

I managed to miss three out of the six meetups, including the graduation ceremony, but I still successfully completed every painting I started.

Preparing for the Process

To prepare for the nine-month-long painting journey, I started taking painting classes at a gallery in Abu Dhabi. My teacher, Lada, was my son's age, had an artist's temperament that worked well with mine, was opinionated, told me what did not work, but also praised my "artistic" solutions to some of the work. She gave me the confidence to continue painting.

DOI: 10.4324/9781003351344-27

Dedicated Space, Time and Resources

Every Monday and Thursday afternoon, I would be sitting at the big table in the inner gallery, with a work in progress or a blank canvas, paints and brushes at the ready for my three hours of painting.

I started getting extra time at the gallery and I became a curiosity, too, with shoppers walking in and around me while I worked. I initially felt intruded upon but soon started enjoying the attention of being watched while I painted. I started believing I was a real artist. I would even take short walks around the mall in my paint-splattered shirts.

Sign Your Work When You Are Done

While in Abu Dhabi, I also attended monthly Corks and Canvas classes at one of the clubs. It was a fun, inspiring acrylic painting activity run by Karissa, who is an artist and photographer.

The room would be laid out with small easels on the table, a custom palette, a picture to copy and canapes at the far end, along with vouchers for two glasses of wine.

At the end of the three hours, we all emerged, well nourished and ready to pose for the traditional group photo of the artists of the day holding up our respective artwork. Every painting was based on the same photo – same colors, same size – yet each painter had her own unique style and came out with a different interpretation of the original picture.

Knowing my tendency to enthusiastically start new projects and lose interest in continuing if the process got too long, I just finished the picture in the allotted time. The manageable 10″ x 8″ to 16″ x 12″ size of the canvas helped me complete it in one session. I had already learned that a painting looks better the next day.

Unresolved Work

Lada, our instructor, left the country suddenly. I had started working on more complicated multimedia projects that were bordering on social activism and needed her guidance. My Color of Woman training had already started, so

I concentrated on that style and kept the "unresolved" canvases aside. Those canvases are still unresolved, as are many new ones I started. But these incomplete pieces weigh less heavily on my conscience as I continue to finish new paintings.

Lessons Learned

The lessons I learned in my first year of formal painting practice include:

1. Get a Buddy, a Coach, a Teacher and/or an Accountability Partner

Forget the "lonely artist" stereotype whenever possible. Humans are social beings and the COVID years have taught us that isolation can be stifling. Still, most creativity is in isolation, giving the very vocal inner critic plenty of time and space to spin her lies. In her own twisted way, the inner critic seems to think that shame is the best motivator. That's not true. We all respond better to appreciation and positive feedback. Don't let anything come between you and your creative work, especially not that pesky inner critic voice.

Work can get done more quickly when you're having fun, chatting, gossiping, sipping something and admiring each other's point of view. Just make an agreement that criticism is not welcome, but helpful suggestions and praise are wonderful for the receiver and the giver. It also helps to make the decision when it's time to put aside the brush, declare the painting is finished and sign it.

Without Lada encouraging me and, from time to time, acknowledging my creative solutions, I would never have finished what I still consider some of my best early work. True, many of them were paintings in the style of Impressionist artists I admire or interpreting other works of art. Any new skill requires practice and imitation, along with acknowledgement, as this is a good way to discover one's own unique style.

Similarly, I completed my earlier Color of Woman 2018 paintings because I was painting alongside far more accomplished artists and with a fixed time frame.

The only time my painting practice stalls is when I am alone in my studio with no one to hold me accountable. That does not say much about my self-discipline muscle, but it says a lot about my need for painting alone together time.

2. Create a Space for Creativity

It is vital for artists to have a dedicated workspace for creativity. Art is a messy business and more so for people who normally create messes whenever they work. When I started painting, I had a studio where I took classes and my house was large enough for me to convert the downstairs bedroom into a studio. When we moved 11,000 kilometers away, my first concern was where I would paint. Fortunately, we found an apartment with a solarium next to the bedroom that was converted into a studio. That is my sacred space.

Your painting space is a place where you spend a lot of time confronting your biases, your beliefs, your weaknesses, your fears and your anxieties and, hopefully, come through it all with some form of resolution. Making art is introspective work. The entire creative process is one in which the end result is not as you imagined it at the beginning. That is a good thing; otherwise, you would not be creating.

3. Three-Hour Time Blocks

There is a reason art classes are scheduled in three-hour blocks. Everything, worthwhile or not, requires the allocation of time. Creativity needs even more time to envision, to sketch, to experiment, to paint, to correct, to remove what's not working and to replace it with what works better.

Painting is organization heavy. It requires material. Brushes need to be washed and the studio needs to be cleaned up and ready for the next session.

It's a good practice to time block at least two three-hour sessions of painting on your calendar per week. Painting daily is even better, but that requires a full commitment to painting and nothing else. In painting, as with many other activities requiring focus and concentration, the process is all encompassing. You cannot paint in short bursts between other activities such as checking the oven, your inbox, or your phone messages (although many people do this and these distractions and avoidances are among the obstacles to completing creative projects).

The natural tendency for many artists is to avoid finding or scheduling the time for painting. The reality is I still paint late at night, when all other activity is completed and long after the 3:00-to-6:00-p.m. time slot. I find this late-night painting isn't healthy as it eats into my sleep and self-care time, but that's how I often complete creative work.

4. Stick to a Set Time Frame for the Project

The projects I finished with minimal drama and avoidance were those that were witnessed or with a definite end-by date to present.

In the summer of 2020, my Red Madonna projects were put on hold. I took a depression break due to political events that have no place in a chapter on completing creative work. Like the rest of my nation, I was completely numb and stayed numb for nearly three months. Yet I had already decided to complete the project. I started and finished two canvases in a week. *The Guardians* (48″ x 60″) represents the events of these challenging times. That painting is a keeper. The other five 36″ x 48″ paintings are part of a larger body of work. I did not sign two of the paintings, thinking they needed rework. As I write this, I realize the project is finished and I'm in a new phase with my creative work.

5. Less Is More

There is such a thing as overworking a project. When you're working alone, give yourself a "wishful" completion time (such as by the end of the month when you start thinking about the project) and a firm deadline. Projects always take more time than you anticipate, but not every idea needs to be included in that one painting.

Be sure to sign your work on the deadline, even if you really hate it. Then put it up on the wall. Examine it from time to time; see what you like or dislike about it. You can also put it away in an "undecided" box. If the feeling persists, recycle the canvas if you can, or use it as a practice board for new ideas. Some unfinished projects were never meant to be finished. Instead, they can be recycled and take on a new life.

Pending work can weigh heavily on the soul until you put it out of sight and out of mind and return to it when you are ready. This summer, I bubble-wrapped all my "unresolved" paintings and put them away in the storeroom to deal with later. My studio now only has three works in progress that need to be finished by year end.

6. Shamelessly Expose Your Work

Show your work at home, gift it to people you trust and when you're feeling comfortable enough, start researching agents and looking for exhibition space. Over time, the canvases build up and you need to redistribute them to create space for your new work. That is something I need to start doing, but I'm kicking that ball forward to 2023.

In the interim, use every opportunity to show off your work. I just show mine to anyone who's interested from the gallery on my phone. The reaction is always good. Maybe they're just polite. But some are genuinely impressed. Most people do not realize how liberating it is to play with paint. Don't get me wrong, I still have a long list of what I can't do. BUT I have managed to slow down the self-deprecation long enough to get into "flow," where I no longer watch the time or judge my work as harshly.

7. Structure and "Intentional Creativity"

I attribute my difficulty with structure to being "creative" and spontaneous. It is a lie I tell myself to avoid the anxiety-provoking planning stage that precedes most work.

I suggest starting with small canvases that can be finished in one or two sessions at most. Smaller paintings are also easier to resolve, improve, store and exhibit.

The intentional creativity process tells stories on larger canvases. The painting and writing are closely related and many practitioners are poets. I am not. I'm still struggling to write and paint together. I record my studio sessions and reflections in multimedia journals to keep track of what's going on.

The blank canvas no longer scares me and the bigger the canvas, the more fun I have. That means I often start more paintings than I finish. So be it. It is all practice, practice, practice until it is completed, signed and exposed.

Over the course of the past five years, since I took up painting seriously, I have also acknowledged that talent alone does not an artist make and the word *mediocre* does not make me cringe the way it did in my 20s. I have always loved art. At first, I was just a collector. Now I'm a painter. Sometimes I get frustrated. I often put off going into the studio and pouring the paints out, but once I do, I love the process and can't get enough of it. Like many artists, I work through the night and burn out during the day. Art and life take on the meaning you give them. The more enjoyable the process, the easier it is to complete your creations.

Three Tips for Creatives

1. Create, create, create. The editor of this book has instilled in us the power of daily practice, preferably first thing in the morning. It works well for writers and larks. Painters and owls may bookend the day with their art. You can only become a professional by working at your craft day in and day out, some days with joy and love, other days less so.
2. It's okay to practice easier, smaller pieces and learn from artists you admire. At the earlier stages, it lets you know when a work is complete. At the later stages, it provides new ways of expressing your own style.
3. Keep on learning and practicing new techniques. Take in-person and group classes whenever possible. They will connect you with others, give you exposure as an artist in progress and prepare you mentally and emotionally for the day when you are the featured artist.

Three Tips for Coaches

1. Be patient with your creative clients. They are highly sensitive to their innate uniqueness, including the shrill sound of their inner critic. As a result, they may be less "coachable," with a slower upward curve.
2. Include relaxation, meditation, breathing and positive-thinking exercises to counter the many mood swings your creative clients might encounter on their long, lonely journey of exposing their work, first to themselves and later to the outside world.
3. Bring them back to their bodies. Creatives spend most of their time in their heads, forgetting that their energy and output is only as good as the container it's in. Daily routines to move – preferably dance – shake, breathe fresh air, eat healthy nourishing meals and sleep well are the secret to better health and greater creativity.

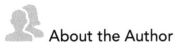 # About the Author

Anni Barsoum is an intentional creativity painter who tells stories that reveal themselves on the canvas. She has been living in Toronto since January 2020, after 35 years of expatriation in the UAE, where she worked in financial services, risk and corporate banking. She discovered her inner painter as an antidote to an empty nest and now sees it as a form of social activism and purposeful living.

How to Get There From Here

28

Using Task Blocks to Complete Your Book

Jude Walsh Whelley

Writers often start off in a blaze of fervor and then bog down. They lose track of the book or are easily distracted by life. So what to do? How do you get "there" from "here?" Task blocks are a writing action plan organized to focus not just on time but on time by task. They help facilitate a solid first draft, then revision and a final close-read edit.

My Story

Some books forever change the way you think. Steven Covey's *7 Habits of Highly Effective People* (1989) affected me that way. Especially Habit #2: Begin With the End in Mind. I began to set goals, fix them in my mind (I was way ahead of the visualization curve) and then start baby-stepping my way toward completion. I love beginnings. As a teacher, the start of every school year found me setting individual goals for each of my students with special needs. There was such satisfaction in checking off completed goals and witnessing their progress.

In 1994, while on a ten-hour interstate drive, I bought a copy of the original *Chicken Soup for the Soul* off a rack of books at a gas station. I read some of the stories aloud to my husband as he drove. We laughed. We cried. Our hearts were touched. I not only loved the stories, but I also loved the book's intention to share inspirational stories that both soothe and comfort readers.

DOI: 10.4324/9781003351344-28

I said, "One day, I'd like to be in a book like this." I had an end in mind, but I did not have a plan to realize that goal. Life intervened and it was many years before I took action on it. I studied the submission rules and began to craft stories. In 2017, my story about one of my students, "Bonus Pay," was published in *Chicken Soup for the Soul: Inspiration for Teachers*.

I experienced a wrenching divorce and wanted to do something to help other women. I had a very specific end in mind. I wanted to write a book that would gather everything I'd learned the hard way into an easy to read guide as traumatized women have difficulty focusing. I wanted it to be small enough to fit in a purse or backpack. I wanted journal prompts to personalize the experience for the reader. I worked with a coach who kept me on task. So, in 2019, I wrote *Post-Divorce Bliss: Ending Us and Finding Me* (Morgan James Press). My positive experience with a coach and my desire to help other women morphed into a coaching practice, working one on one with clients using my book as a guide.

Writing personal essays and self-help came easily to me. When I began to write fiction, I struggled with how to get the book done. I needed to have an end in mind and I needed a plan, defined steps and strategies to get there. And I was not alone. I found one strategy – using task blocks – particularly helpful. Now much of my work is with writers. I offer short-term coaching to help writers establish a creative practice that supports their dream, along with helping them master techniques and strategies to complete their work.

Coaching

The task-block strategy that was most helpful for my own writing is now a staple in my coaching practice. It is a variation on the Pomodoro method of timed writing. *Pomodoro* is the Italian word for *tomato*. Francesco Cirillo developed the strategy of setting a timer and writing until the timer went off. The timer he used was shaped like a tomato: hence, the Pomodoro method. Writers can find these timed sessions, usually referred to as Writing Sprints, on the Internet.

I learned the task-block variation from author and coach Sarra Cannon. Instead of using time as the sole indicator, work is focused on measurable tasks. Task blocks use timing as well, usually twenty-five minutes, allowing for two task blocks in an hour, with two five-minute breaks. The difference is that the work is planned by task, as opposed to being organized simply around time.

Beginning with the end – a completed novel – in mind, let's walk through the three stages to book completion – first draft, revision and editing – and apply the task-block strategy to each. First, decide what you want to achieve, figure out how to measure that and then match that measure to a time block.

First draft: let's say that your goal is a 75,000-word first draft of a novel. Write for twenty-five minutes and then count your words. Do that several times and then average your word counts. For ease of example, let's say you write an average of 500 words in twenty-five minutes. Divide 75,000 words by 500 and you can see you need 150 twenty-five minute time blocks to reach your goal. Add an extra 10% to give some ease. So plan for 165 task blocks, or 82.5 hours. That covers task blocks for the first draft, but to complete a book, you also need time for revision and editing.

Revision: how to quantify a block in revision? Word count is no longer as good a measure as you are going to be both removing and adding words. It is easier to go by pages. A common page estimate is 250 words per page, so a 75,000-word book is 300 pages. Set a timer for 25 minutes and see how many pages you can revise. This varies widely, depending on the status of the manuscript. A first revision might be slow going; a second pass through might be a bit faster. For purposes of this example, let's say that it turns out that you manage 10 pages in 25 minutes. So you would plan for 30 25-minute task blocks for revision – 15 hours – with a 1.5-hour, 10% buffer, which amounts to 16.5 hours for revision.

Editing: this is a close look at a manuscript, checking for typos, punctuation errors and consistent formatting. Some writers find it hard to edit their own work. It is almost always a good idea to have fresh eyes do this pass if possible. One way to do it yourself is to use the read-oud feature from your software. Listen for twenty-five minutes and see how many pages have been read. Use that as your baseline. Follow the manuscript, looking for errors as it is read aloud. You will definitely need a break after twenty-five minutes. You may even want to modify the time period if twenty-five minutes is too fatiguing. Let's estimate seven to eight hours.

We have now determined that to get this book completed to the point where it could go to a beta reader or to a critique group, you need 107 (82.5 + 16.5 + 8) hours of dedicated task blocks. In addition to having a good estimate of how many task blocks are needed, you also need a realistic estimate of how much time you have available (your schedule) and how many hours in a row you can work (your endurance) in a week. Take into consideration work and family obligations as well as some self-care. Then slot task blocks into your available time and you have the number of weeks needed to complete the tasks necessary to finish your book. You've gone from here to there.

Three Tips for Creatives

1. Plan some fun into this. Maybe make a silly sticker chart to track completed blocks. Have special snacks ready for those five-minute breaks. Set special rewards at certain intervals: a Netflix binge between stages, a special smoothie or cocktail every 20 blocks, a hike, or a dinner out.

2. Know your fatigue factor. Keep track of your project and make some notes as to what is effective for you and when. For example, you may know that when writing a first draft, the writing is fast and furious, so plan on more words per block for then. If doing a developmental write, that may take more thought and, therefore, be more demanding. When doing the first draft, you might easily do block sessions twice a day. Developmental work may fatigue you more easily and when you're fatigued, productivity decreases. Better to have two productive hours than four hours with diminishing returns.

3. Hold fast to the end goal. Post it on your mirror so it is the first thing you see in the morning. Tape it to your computer. Do a vision board featuring your book. Make a cover mock-up and frame it for your desk. Take a few minutes every day to imagine how good this will feel when complete.

 Three Tips for Coaches

1. Once the goal has been established, coach your client first to see the stages (first draft, revision, editing) and then to quantify the stage work into tasks.

2. Use a scaffolding approach. Provide a high level of assistance at the beginning of each stage and then gradually withdraw, encouraging the client to employ the technique without your assistance.

3. Ask your client to share progress: task block completions as well as transitions to the next stage. Send occasional encouraging texts or emails. A simple shared chart, like a Google Doc, will let you see progress so you can respond in a timely manner.

Recommended Resources:

The 7 Habits of Highly Effective People (Steven R. Covey)
The Pomodoro Technique (Francesco Cirillo)
Chicken Soup for the Soul (Jack Canfield and Mark Victor Hansen)
Sarra Cannon, author and coach at Heart Breathings (www.youtube.com/ heartbreathings)

 ## About the Author

Jude Walsh Whelley is a creativity and mindset coach and the author of *Post-Divorce Bliss: Ending Us and Finding Me* (Morgan James Press 2019). She's published in numerous anthologies and literary magazines and is currently completing her first novel. Jude coaches women post-divorce and writers wanting to establish creative practice habits and routines.

Finishing by Design   **29**

Jamie Palmer

Finishing. It can be a dirty word for creatives. How many of us creatives have a pile of long-lost projects that we started and never finished? For me, it's more than I'd like to admit. The reality is that unfinished work is synonymous with doing creative work. My role as a coach is to support clients in shifting their relationship with finishing. Far too many times, I have witnessed client after client give themselves head trash over why they didn't finish, rationalizing it, overexplaining it and using excuses. Yet these excuses only prolong finishing.

As a human design business coach supporting entrepreneurs for the last 19 years, I have noticed common themes around why creatives don't finish. I call these "your finishing designs." The five most common finishing designs and their voices are:

1. Glittery object syndrome – "Oh, look! This will be the thing that changes the game."
2. Perfectionism – "I'm just going to tweak this and that," which gets repeated and repeated.
3. Mismatched expectations – "I thought I'd be able to get this done in X amount of time, but it is going to take far longer."
4. No momentum – "I can't get back into flow to bring the project to the finish line."
5. Passion is gone – "I got into the project and realized that I hate it."

Anytime I see clients struggle to finish, it is a clear red flag to me that they are telling themselves a story about why they can't finish. This story is often a fear response. Our brains keep us safe. Creative work requires a level of vulnerability and transparency. When we create, we share a piece of ourselves, our soul, with the world. It is innately personal and intimate. Yet we compound the struggle to finish with negative self-talk, further prolonging the finishing process.

DOI: 10.4324/9781003351344-29

Ultimately, to reckon with this "story," it becomes imperative first to recognize that we are telling ourselves a story. I like the metaphor of a penalty flag on the field, like in American football. Are we aware that a penalty flag is sending us a clear signal that we have a project to finish, but we are feeding ourselves an excuse? The sooner we recognize that flag on the creative playing field, the sooner we can tend to the story we are telling ourselves and finish.

Once we become aware that we are telling ourselves a story, we must then discern where this story is coming from. What is it keeping us safe from? What lesson do we need to learn from this? How can we write a new story? We must get to the root of why we aren't finishing to embrace a new story so that we can finish.

I worked with a client on her book and book launch a few years ago. Every time we would get close to launching, she would self-sabotage by purchasing another program or course, then stalling to incorporate this "new thing": a.k.a. glittery object syndrome. She repeatedly told me, "I just know this will be the thing that changes the game of my launch." The red flag was on her creative field.

After the third time, we discussed her pattern of not finishing her book launch and fully committing to a strategy. I asked her to journal and reflect on what she believed was holding her back. Where had that come from in her life? Was there a time in her childhood when that served her well?

After a few days of going back and forth, she recalled a time in her childhood when a teacher gave her detention for turning in a paper early. She recalled how devastating this experience was. She even remembered vowing to herself she would never "get stuff done early ever again."

This client's glittery object syndrome story was keeping her safe. However, this glittery object syndrome was no longer serving her need to finish projects. It was time to rewrite the story.

When we enter the act of creative work, it is by design an act of radical vulnerability. While we might not think of it that way, creative work is the unique expression of our being, our synthesis and who we are. Our work, whether written or visual, is on display for the world to experience. Perhaps they will love it. Maybe they will hate it.

We have no objective evidence of what others will think. When we release our creative work into the world, we expose ourselves to judgment, criticism and feedback. We humans want to be accepted into our community for who we are. Rejection is one of our primal fears. This fear of rejection and criticism can prevent us from finishing work on a subconscious level.

This subconscious fear presents itself as procrastination and excuses around why we can't finish. These excuses include glittery object syndrome, perfectionism, overcommitment, no passion, mismatched expectations, etc. Getting to the root of the reason requires us to look at what story we are telling ourselves about why we cannot finish.

I tend to fall into the category of mismatched expectations and perfectionism. Different iterations of these excuses played out in various forms throughout the years, particularly with my writing. I would sit on a piece of writing for months, tweaking and tweaking but never completing it. I often asked myself, "Who would want to read what I wrote anyway?"

After reflecting on why I believed this, I recalled being rejected in high school for a national poetry award. When I dug deeper, through journaling and mindful exercises, I remembered that my guidance counselor had told me, "If you want a career as a writer, be prepared to struggle." This was not necessarily true, but it kept me from doing the vulnerable work of putting my creative work out into the world. To finish creative work, we must reckon with the limiting beliefs that hold us back. We must learn to dance with them instead of fighting against them. We must befriend them. We must tend to them to finish our creative work. Otherwise, they will keep us stuck.

With an awareness of the voices that hold us back from finishing, we can begin to shine a light on where we might struggle to finish. We can recognize more quickly when there is a penalty flag on our creative field of play. We can show ourselves compassion and understanding instead of negative self-talk. We can tend to the excuses and uncover the story beneath them. We can get clear on how to finish by design.

 Three Tips for Creatives

1. Take regular breaks from your work to do something else. Spend time in nature, connect with friends, or simply do nothing. Taking time out from your work helps you gain new perspectives and innovation.
2. Recognize when you have a flag on your creative field. What excuses are you telling yourself about finishing your work?
3. Create a folder on your computer of all the compliments people have given you about your work. When you are questioning yourself about finishing your work, pull up this content and remind yourself of your contribution.

Three Tips for Coaches

1. Begin to notice and recognize which finishing designs and sayings are emerging in the stories you are telling yourself. Write them down.
2. Step away from your work. Slow down, get present and be grounded. Reflect on the story you are telling yourself. Are there any consistent patterns? How is that story serving you? Or not? Where did it come from? Do you have evidence for or against it? What would it look like to let that story go? What lesson do you want to carry forward? Journal or take an intentional walk to reflect on these questions.
3. What story do you need to let go of to finish? Thank yourself for the lesson. Keep a log or journal with evidence of the positive things that happen when you finish.

 ## About the Author

Jamie Palmer is a human design expert with a difference. With a unique ability to take a hawk's-eye view and her fearless need to explore the depths and evolve, Jamie is on a mission to innovate and liberate you from the false beliefs and obstacles that hold you back in your life and biz. Jamie believes your voice is essential to a future in which we can thrive, not only as individuals but also connected to the beauty of a sustainable ecosystem. Jamie lives in Newport, RI, with her kiddos and husband, hanging out in nature, paddleboarding, or turning her backyard into an edible landscape.

Factoring In the Impact of Your Creative Work

30

Danielle Langin

As creatives, we have a responsibility to complete projects that bring value, change, purpose and beauty to the world. This chapter is about feeling into this responsibility and factoring in the impact as it pertains to your current creative project. Through examples, guidance and prompts for reflection, you will gain clarity around the value of your work, how people will benefit from your work and the impact it will have as a whole once it's completed. Doing so will inspire you to keep up the momentum, all the while offering you a deeper understanding of the way your creativity leaves a mark on those on the receiving end, a piece that is so often missing in the process of bringing a project from start to finish.

What Does It Mean to Have an Impact?

By its most simple definition, to have an impact is to have a strong effect on someone or something. But let's expand on this a bit more. To have an impact isn't just to affect someone or something; it's to influence, to touch, to change, to alter and to potentially pull that someone or something in a direction they weren't heading before. We'll dive deeper into what impact actually looks like, but essentially, especially in the creative world, to have an impact is to inspire change, pique curiosity, or cultivate a sense of beauty for those on the receiving end.

DOI: 10.4324/9781003351344-30

The Impact of Creativity and the Arts

Creativity is a mirror and a powerful reflector, so we shouldn't underestimate the impact our creative work may have on ourselves, those around us and society as a whole. Like a ripple effect, our work can create powerful waves of change, inspiration, beauty, conversation, depth, purpose, motivation, discovery and joy in our own community and beyond.

It's the way your finished painting brings joy to a room. It's the way your finished song allows a hurting person to begin the process of healing. It's the way your finished book motivates another writer to write or a person who feels lost to take steps forward or an artist to finish their creative work and so on.

Art has this effect. Art has this ability. This is something we already deeply understand as creatives and something we must be willing to factor into the importance of completing our own projects.

Consider this book and its chapters. Each one has been carefully crafted and thoughtfully pieced together with the hope of encouraging its readers to complete their creative work. This was the intention: to inspire, motivate and encourage creative readers like yourself to finish a project they set out to do despite the internal and external obstacles that may arise in the process. The impact is what you, the reader, take away from it. How will reading this book affect your life? How will it influence the ways in which you approach your creative process? How will it alter your perspective, inspire change and emotionally empower you toward completing your creative work?

These are the questions we must ask ourselves as creatives who are bringing art, poetry and expression to the world, especially when we are nearing the finish line for a creative endeavor. What will the impact be? Who will this art touch and how will it change their lives?

The Ways Creativity Creates Impact

Here are some of the ways a creative project, whether it be a painting, a mural, a book of poetry, a song, or a self-help book, can create lasting impact. See if you can add to this list based on your own experiences or the experiences of people around you.

Creative projects can affect ourselves and others by:

- Cultivating joy
- Inspiring, motivating and encouraging change
- Making beauty out of the mundane

- Inviting depth into conversations
- Eliciting an emotional response
- Supporting reflection and contemplation
- Giving a sense of purpose and meaning
- Aiding in self-discovery

Challenges You May Come Up Against

As with any obstacle on the creative path, you may find yourself coming up against specific challenges with regard to seeing the value of your creative work. The thoughts and feelings around these challenges can sound like this:

- "Who am I to complete this project?"
- "I'm afraid to complete this project."
- "I'm not good enough to complete this project."
- "No one will like what I create."
- "No one will care about what I create."
- "Nothing I create is worthy of finishing."

When these thoughts arise is when the real work comes in around being a creative person. Not only do we have an opportunity to coach ourselves and do the deep inner work of overcoming our creative blocks, but we also have the opportunity to understand the value of our creative project and the ways it will leave a mark on ourselves and others.

Again, ask yourself, "What will the impact of my creative work be? What kind of response will it elicit? Who will benefit from this project and why?"

You may find it helpful to do a visualization exercise along with some journaling exercises to build the muscle of being able to recognize the worth your creative work carries.

Visualizing the Impact of Your Creative Work

One of the biggest creative projects I've worked on was a deck of journal prompt cards called *The Flowers Within*. The inspiration for the project was strong and motivating until it wasn't and all the work I had done was left completely untouched in a corner of a room for over a year.

To inspire myself to finish the deck, I sat in my meditation corner and closed my eyes. I envisioned what it would be like to bring this deck to life, how I would feel when it was finished and how people would receive the deck and use it.

In my visualization, I imagined that the people using this deck would grow a more beautiful relationship with their writing. I imagined the ways my deck would change, inspire and impact their lives. I allowed every detail of what the journey would be like for the people on the receiving end once I finished the project and hit publish.

When I was done with my visualization, I journaled on the experience, taking note of the value, importance and purpose I felt this deck would bring to people.

This moment of solitude and reflection lit the creative spark in me again and I was able to complete the project and publish it. The best part is I still get messages to this day from people sharing the ways the deck has helped them, just as I envisioned.

Try a similar visualization exercise for yourself about your own creative work the next time you feel stalled or stuck.

Creating Space for Self-Reflection

Next time you are stuck in the middle phase of a creative project and are unsure how to gain momentum to finish it, create the space for reflection and journal on the following questions:

1. Why does the world need my current creative work?
2. Who will benefit from my current creative work?
3. In what ways will they benefit?
4. Are there ways my current creative work will inspire, motivate, encourage, or move the person/people on the receiving end? If so, in what ways?
5. Why do I *really* need to complete this project?
6. How will this completed project affect my own life as well as the lives of others?
7. What is it about my unique creative approach to this project that will give it even more value and allow for more impact?

 Three Tips for Creatives

1. Bring a sense of reflection and curiosity to your creative project. Continue the process of asking yourself questions related to the

value and impact of this project and what it will bring to the table. Continuing this internal dialogue will aid you when you come up against obstacles.

2. Give yourself the space to work through your blocks as they arise. With any creative project you are working on, you are going to feel a variety of feelings from excitement and inspiration to fear and self-criticism. Allow yourself to feel the entirety of the process and get support where it is needed.

3. On the flip side of this, practice discipline and take action. While it's important to give your creative self enough space to reflect, it's equally important to show up with dedication and determination so that you can finish your project.

Three Tips for Coaches

1. Work with your clients on their self-worth as a creative. They can't factor in the impact of their creative work if they don't see the value in what they are creating or their value as a creative person.

2. Mirror back to your client the value you see in their creative project. Is there an importance, a purpose, an impact and/or a reason that comes to mind when they tell you of their project? If so, share this with them and see if they can begin to see it too.

3. Explore with a client what the impact may be of their finished project. Remember to invite them to explore the impact it will have not only on others but also on themselves and their lives. Feel free to use the journal prompts in this chapter to help them go deeper in their reflection.

Remember, creativity is needed in this world. Whether you're creating a deck of cards, a book, a painting, an album, or a song, there is a place in this world for your work. The project you are breathing to life has a reason to exist and be completed and it will leave an impact deeper than you can possibly imagine. Don't forget to factor in this impact and, more importantly, the impact it will have on you if you don't.

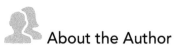 ## About the Author

Danielle Langin is a writer, poet, creativity coach and certified Journal to the Self instructor. She believes that the more we create, the more we heal and because of this, her work is deeply rooted in mindfulness and self-reflection. You can find her on Instagram @daniellelangin or visit her website, http://daniellelangin.com.

Timely Completing via Right Thinking

31

Eric Maisel

The central premise of cognitive therapy is that wrong thinking causes much of the pain and suffering we experience. The Roman Epictetus put it this way: "Do not surrender your mind." Wise men and wise woman have informed us since the dawn of our species that we are what we think. If what you are thinking supports not completing your creative projects, you won't complete them.

Wrong thinking produces pain and suffering. The antidote is right thinking. The Buddha said, "Get a grip on your mind!" As a thoughtful person, you have the ability to challenge thoughts that bring you pain or prevent you from completing your creative projects. What you also need are the understanding and the will. If you have the understanding and the will, then when a wrong thought pops into your head, you will see it clearly for what it is: the product of some doubt, fear, reluctance, or inner conflict and you will instantly and forthrightly deal with it.

The first step is clearly hearing the thought and recognizing it for what it is. The next step is saying, "I don't want this thought!" In cognitive therapy, this is called thought confrontation. Without hesitation and without embarrassment, you say "No!" The final step is to replace the unbidden, unfortunate thought with a right thought. In cognitive therapy, this is called thought substitution. With the right thought in place, the pain ends.

At a writers' conference, a writer asked me, "Can I really do that? Can I get rid of thoughts I've been thinking my whole life and replace them with new ones?" I replied, "If you want to." That is the complete answer. You may not want to for one or another of a hundred different reasons. In that case, you won't. You will keep your current thoughts and all the pain and suffering they engender. And your creative projects will remain unfinished.

DOI: 10.4324/9781003351344-31

The goal of this work is not to become a Pollyanna. You do not replace wrong thoughts with happy thoughts. You replace them with affirmative thoughts that are full of true understanding and an appreciation of reality. You do not replace "I can never write my novel" with "If I sing a happy tune, I can write my novel in three days flat!" You do not replace "No one will publish my collection of poems" with "Everyone will want to publish my collection of poems!" You replace the first with "I can write my novel" and the second with "I will do a terrific job of marketing my collection, the best job I can possibly do." Those are the sorts of affirmations and thought substitutes you want to entertain.

Maybe we won't do a perfect job of preventing wrong thinking from infiltrating our consciousness, noticing it when it occurs, or instantly introducing right thinking to counteract our wrong thoughts. But we can get much better at all three. I train creativity coaches and we discuss these issues. One creativity coach in training shared the following anecdote. This is an excellent and, I hope, inspiring example of how far we can come.

> This week, I caught myself in a thought that surprised me. I'm sitting on my bed with a drawing pad across my lap charting chunks of my novel. Five or six large pages, vivid with ovals and arrows, spill across the bed and onto the floor. For weeks, I'd been feeling pleased that my current mix of characters and events have attracted a strong flow, especially since not having enough material had been an old fear. I'd been lucky to strike a gusher. So, who is this saying: "You know how you overcomplicate things. Keep it simple, can't you?"

> I didn't notice this commentary at first. I'd been intent on what I was doing and believed I was enjoying the process when I started to feel a dark mood, rather like what happens in a science fiction movie when an alien space ship casts a giant shadow over a city. I wanted to shoo it away. Then I finally noticed the words I'd been hearing. I've had lots of experience at counteracting blurts, so I didn't stop to analyze. Instantly, I treated myself to a positive affirmation and printed it at the top of the page I'd been working on. Right mind: "You have wonderfully rich resources to draw upon." The space ship withdrew and I happily filled another eight or so pages, printing the positive thought at the top of each page.

My hope is that you can learn to think right, in general and specifically when it comes to completing your creative projects. I hope you can learn to say, "I am writing today," instead of "I am so tired." I hope you can learn to say, "I wrote a first novel and now I'm starting on my second novel," instead of "I wrote an awful first novel and that proves I'm an idiot." Neither you nor I can answer any of the ultimate questions. But don't you feel at least a little confident that you can substitute a right thought for a wrong thought? If you're convinced that the answer is no, opt for yes anyway. Unless you opt to say yes to the possibility that you can change your mind and with it your life, you will have said no with a vengeance.

You may not be very clear on what wrong thinking and right thinking sound like. Therefore, I want to provide you some pairs of wrong thoughts and right thoughts so that you will become super clear on the difference between a wrong thought and a right thought. By "wrong," I mean a thought that doesn't serve you. A thought may be true and still not serve you and if it doesn't serve you, then it is a wrong thought for you to be countenancing, even though it is true. Many true thoughts do not serve us, especially as we try to finish our creative projects! Is it useful to have thoughts circulating in your brain about a famine in Africa, the demise of brick-and-mortar book-stores, how few songs you've produced over the past year, or that your mother is ailing as you try to finish the last song for your musical comedy? All these fall into the category of "Not now, thought!"

Here are ten pairs of wrong thoughts and right thoughts, presented from a writer's point of view. I know that you'll be able to translate them into whatever artistic genre you work in. Please begin to see how the second of each pair is so much better for you to be thinking than the first! If you regularly think the first, you will have tremendous trouble completing your creative projects. If you regularly think the second, you will get your creative project completed.

1. Wrong mind: "I am a stupid, neurotic person with no real talent. I don't really matter."
   Right mind: "I matter."
2. Wrong mind: "In some important sense, I am ruined."
   Right mind: "Many wounded people have written. I can be a wounded writer. Maybe I can even become a healed writer."
3. Wrong mind: "There is far too much going on in my life for me to write."
   Right mind: "I will write first thing every morning."
4. Wrong mind: "My to-do list is so full, there is no room on it for writing."
   Right mind: "Writing is at the top of my to-do list."
5. Wrong mind: "My mind is so noisy that I can't think straight."
   Right mind: "I can quiet my mind just by saying, 'Hush.'"
6. Wrong mind: "I hate mistakes and messes."
   Right mind: "I am easy with mistakes and messes."

7. Wrong mind: "I can't write when the temperature is below 68 degrees or above 72 degrees."

   Right mind: "I can write in a thunderstorm by the light of lightning bolts."

8. Wrong mind: "I will definitely get back to my novel next week."

   Right mind: "Ready or not, I am heading to the computer."

9. Wrong mind: "I can't write if I outline. Outlining kills the creative spark in me."

   Right mind: "I can write with an outline and I can write without an outline. I can even write in the shower with a bar of soap."

10. Wrong mind: "I can't write without an outline. If I don't have an outline, I meander all over the place and end up in Bulgaria."

    Right mind: "I can write with an outline and I can write without an outline. I can even write standing on my head, until I pass out."

 Three Tips for Creatives

1. Believe that you can get a grip of your own mind. Then actually get that grip!
2. Begin to recognize the ways that thoughts aren't serving you. When you notice a thought that isn't serving you, dispute it and substitute a more useful thought.
3. Pay particular attention to your thoughts as you near the end of a creative project!

 Three Tips for Coaches

1. When you hear a client say something that you have the sense isn't serving them, bring that to their attention. You might phrase it as follows: "I wonder, do you think what you just said is serving you?"
2. Whether or not you officially do cognitive therapy, create your ways of working "cognitively" with clients as they need that help!
3. Check out you own self-talk. How much of it is serving you? Maybe you'd like to do a little disputing and substituting yourself!

About the Author

Eric Maisel is the author of 50+ books. His recent books include *Why Smart Teens Hurt, Redesign Your Mind* and *The Power of Daily Practice*. Among his other books are *Coaching the Artist Within, Fearless Creating, Rethinking Depression* and *The Van Gogh Blues*. Dr. Maisel writes the *Rethinking Mental Health* blog for *Psychology Today*, with 3,000,000+ views and is the creator and lead editor for the Ethics International Press Critical Psychology and Critical Series. A retired family therapist and active creativity coach, Dr. Maisel's forthcoming books include *The Coach's Way* (New World Library) and *Deconstructing ADHD* (Ethics International Press). Dr. Maisel provides workshops, webinars and keynotes nationally and internationally; trains creativity coaches; and facilitates support groups for writers. You can visit him at www.ericmaisel. com and contact him at ericmaisel@hotmail.com.

Mind Yourself   **32**

Nicky Peters

Completing a creative project is much the same as completing a life project –
how you do one is invariably how you do the other. Since we are creatures of
habit, it is likely that your unique pattern of behavior subconsciously deter-
mines almost every part of your life. See if you can identify yourself in one of
the following scenarios:

- You tend to quit at the first hurdle no matter the loss.
- You settle for less since it's unlikely that better exists.
- You procrastinate so much that the end is more a relief than a celebratory
  win.
- Your projects stay trapped in your anguished conscious, never to make it
  out alive.

Of course, there's a reason why your endeavors fail to achieve their intended
result So, let's have a look at what these might be.

Beforehand, let's first understand that environmental factors are the least
likely cause. If you direct blame outside yourself, you forfeit your responsibility to the process. Giving external factors more power than they deserve is
simply your mind's way of preventing you from getting what you want for
fear of what will happen. And as humans, we love abdicating responsibility.
Believing that you gave your best effort despite the odds or that the situation
was out of your control is tempting and reassuring yet entirely disempowering. What message are you telling yourself by doing so?

Mind is perched somewhere abstract in the core of your being and deter-
mines almost every single detail of your life. The degree to which it influences
you is determined by how much you can and know how to dialogue with it. It
is not a one-way set of instructions but a relationship needing good communication. When you embrace dialogue with Mind, you form an alliance and
enter productively alongside it into the creative structure.

DOI: 10.4324/9781003351344-32

Creative Structure

This refers to how you create everything that exists in your life, from the illustrious career (or not) to the birth of an artistic project or your reaction to any given situation. You are constantly creating, even if you are unaware of it. Though much creation is done passively, there are often times when you try to bring something to life. This is, however, when Mind usually gets involved, forever fervent in its mission to protect you at the expense of your creations. This happens by way of one of the following three exits out of the creative structure: **impatience, comparison and abandonment**.

The reasons you might prioritize any one of these exits over completing a project are the result of subconscious beliefs that you hold about yourself and the world around you. These, you most likely created during your childhood, when you had very little experience to draw from. Would you let a small child make all your decisions for you? Undoubtedly not, yet this is largely what you do when you don't address your subconscious beliefs. So what might this look like?

Try to identify yourself in one of the following scenarios:

- You eagerly started an online course during the COVID confinement, but your interest waned a third of the way through. It seemed great at first, but then, frustrated by your progress, you prioritized other tasks. This is **impatience**. It shows up as small yet persuasive excuses for why results are not forthcoming, creating a mental distance between you and your intended result until you eventually abandon it. Ask yourself why.
- People have said that your side hustle is unique and impressive and could earn you an income. But then you discover an established competitor offers a better service and decide that you could never be successful while they are in business. This is **comparison**. It is usually based on inaccurate perceptions of reality, which allow you to avoid the dangers of risk-taking while remaining safely unaccomplished. Ask yourself why.
- You have an unfinished painting that once pulled you into the creative flow but is now collecting dust in the corner of the room. You thrived at the easel but soon stopped going there, fearful of ruining it. This is **abandonment**. Doubt convinces you to abandon your dreams as Mind doesn't want you to be skilled, fulfilled, or successful. Ask yourself why.

Yet let's not portray Mind as all negative, for it is your biggest supporter. Mind was there when you were little, defining your world when you were desperately trying to get oriented. It created your beliefs to protect, prioritize, or benefit you in some way to enable your survival in a confusing and unexplained world. United by a common interest, however, which is your ongoing existence, Mind and you make the perfect pair. Taking back control of the stories you construct your life with is not only possible but inevitable if you commit to getting an accurate view of your reality. Do this by considering more perspectives and identifying what becomes obvious. Of course, this is simple but not easy.

Psychological versus Creative Tension

Since we've looked at what holds you back in the creative structure, now let's focus on what moves you forward. Here, we discover a battle between creative tension and psychological tension. When psychological tension wins, it shows as one of the previously mentioned exits: **impatience, comparison, or abandonment**. Yet when creative tension wins, concepts and ideas take on a physical form in the physical world. Your creative tension is the strength of your desire to produce a work of art, effect conscious change, or masterfully manage life's daily dramas. Think of creative tension as the life force within you, the quiet witness that influences your decision-making in favor of what you love. It's the power of your dreams, the strength of your most wanted feelings, that yearning for different ways of being or experiencing and the part of you that wishes to be expressed to its fullest.

To complete any project, your creative tension must outweigh all life's obstacles and Mind's traps and it must do this right to the glorious end. Since this is not easily achieved, you can improve your chances of succeeding by accessing Mind, either consciously or through hypnosis.

Hypnotherapy for Resolving Psychological Tension

Hypnotherapy has long been considered one of the most effective ways of communicating with Mind's hidden depths. It's an intriguing path of discovery into what stunts your natural perfect functioning and creative tension building. While the conscious mind is temporarily tucked away, Mind can receive healing for past damage to the psyche and establish healthier coping strategies through suggestion. New strategies replace the old ones that Mind once invented as solutions to previous problems, also removing any secondary effects created by the previous strategy. This gives Mind a way to maintain its positive intention toward you but liberates you from the tension caused by outdated strategies or solutions.

Observing the conflict between creative and psychological tensions in a hypnotherapy session provides insight into the individual's challenge without the bias and attempted reasoning of the active consciousness. In the following examples, three artists struggle with the concept of completion. They each demonstrate their unique approach to leaving and subsequently returning to the creative structure.

Three Artists Struggle With the Concept of Completion

Ida

Ida, 43 years old, from Finland, arrives at the session presenting with procrastination. She is a visual artist and the mother of two boys who struggles with lacking confidence and low self-esteem.

Under hypnosis, Ida's Mind reveals that her procrastination keeps her alive. As a child, her jealous mother, among others, would attack her whenever she attempted to "bring joy into the world": a metaphor interpreted by Ida to mean her art. Ida's conscious Mind now allows her to express her creativity, but doubt forces her to abandon it because of the risk of danger. She suggests the solution of better self-care to support herself and consequently attract more supportive, motivating people into her life so she can release her creations into the world safely.

Effectively communicating with Ida's Mind requires a wide visual vocabulary with adjectives and expressions to help her successfully envision her desired transformation. Her metaphor of "lead wolf" represents her as a Nordic creature fearlessly, lovingly leading herself and her pack (her children and her art) more fiercely out into the wild (her environment).

This metaphor strengthens her creative tension in favor of her desired results – to become the fearless leader of both her human and artistic creations so they may exist one day independently of her. Her suggestion of better self-care reduces her psychological tension by meeting her Mind's needs in a healthier way. With more balanced tensions, Ida is better equipped and mentally adapted in her artistic pursuit to complete the projects that she had not previously been able to.

Mary

Mary, 52 years old, from Australia, is an artist and musician who presents with fear of failure and resistance to promoting her artwork and podcast series. Now in the launch stage of her creations, she feels overwhelmed "putting herself out there" and easily discouraged by naysayers online.

In her session, Mary discovers the belief that her art will never be successful since neither she nor her talent was respected by others during her adolescence. At the time, Mary identified herself as a failure in comparison to her sisters. She decided that any positive recognition for her artwork was an isolated incident and not anything she could naturally recreate. She also doubted her ability to make an artistic career sustainable, seemingly reinforced years later by the closure of her art gallery.

Yet far from reinforcing this so-called truth, the gallery's closure reinforced a lifelong strategy of self-doubt, which served to protect her from future rejection. When you subconsciously choose to accept a belief, your Mind always looks for ways to confirm it. This is confirmation bias and it's a means of orientation to increase chances of survival at the expense of logic and a balanced view of the situation. Mary would reject any evidence of her real capabilities when it didn't correspond to her long-held negative self-bias.

Predominantly auditory and kinesthetic, the vocabulary of sound and words that convey motion are best for communicating with Mary's Mind. She wishes to start projects with a "big bang" and decides to listen to frequency-healing music on a regular basis. She reframes her original metaphor of failure through the art gallery's closure to now represent the opposite: her success. That she had managed to create an art gallery would now be proof of her capability. Since she'd done it once, there would be nothing stopping her from doing it again with more patience and the benefit of lessons previously learned.

Katy

Katy, 40 years old, from the UK, is a sensitive artist and mother of two girls, presenting with procrastination, self-sabotage, anxiety and a tendency to abandon projects when near completion.

During her session, Katy discovers that her problems are a side effect of cripplingly low self-esteem triggering extreme alertness designed to avoid creating confrontation with her abusive father. Consequently, doubt and fear prevent her from most activities that could invite danger, since her Mind now sees the world with abuse waiting to happen around every corner.

Highly kinesthetic, Katy describes the world with weighted emphasis on movement, thoughts and feelings. She wishes to feel hopeful and not allow her passions to "grind to a halt." She desires stability and, most importantly, to feel confident "pulling the trigger" when it's time to complete creative projects. Emotive vocabulary that conveys energy and power works best for changing her critical self-talk and she reframes her sensitivity as a force of strength in her exploration of the unknown, with her intuitive feelers as her superpower. She decides that her sensitive autopilot will not only advance her further into the creative structure but also will now make her "unstoppable."

Here, Katy now uses evidence that once worked against her as evidence in her favor. This change of perception opens her up to a more accurate view of reality so that faith might replace doubt in controlling her behavior and prevent her from abandoning any potential joy in her life.

Mind Your Focus

Staying in the creative structure to the point of completion sends a clear message to your subconscious that you are a powerful creator and can have and experience whatever it is that you want. Inevitably, however, the opposite of this is equally true. Abandonment reinforces the belief that you are powerless and will never have what you desire. More the reason to avoid it. Had Mary waited longer and tried out new approaches to her gallery business instead of throwing in the towel, might her gallery have survived the first time around? The temptation to withdraw when things appear not to be working is often too enticing to resist. Additionally, unfair comparison and self-doubt can run rampant through negative self-talk. This encourages you to focus on your psychological tension instead of all the possibilities that are likely to present themselves when you focus instead on your creative tension.

Completing the creative structure can be effortless as long as you place your focus in the right direction and are disciplined enough to hold it there for a given time. Bravely putting yourself out there to publish your first book, sell your artwork, or make your current relationship a resounding success represents an accumulation of all your efforts up to that moment. This act holds the compounding pressures of each expectation, failure and reward, that occurred along the way. So how better to value your life and those who live it with you than by seeing projects through to the end? Of course, whether you are successful or not is determined by the winning tension. And this is ultimately for you to decide. Or Mind will do it for you.

Three Tips for Creatives

1. Get an accurate view of your current reality to avoid negative self-confirmation bias. Ask others to help you see the elements of your situation differently and reframe stories of supposed failure as stories of learning that get you closer to your goal.
2. Question the small yet persuasive excuses with which you reassure yourself that leaving the creative structure is the right thing to do. Remember that impatience, comparison and self-doubt are really symptoms of underlying psychological tension.
3. Focus on what you want to create, what it would feel like and all the reasons you want to create it. Don't worry about how it will materialize; just maintain the belief that it will.

 Three Tips for Coaches

1. Encourage your clients to write down all the beliefs that they hold to be true around a particular situation. During the session, discuss each one to gauge its validity to help your client develop a more accurate view of their reality.
2. To build rapport and develop trust, identify if a client is visual, auditory, or kinesthetic. This gives you clues as to how they perceive and experience the world and can offer tools to help resolve their psychological tension.
3. Look out for metaphors that clients use when describing their situations. Metaphors are a powerful way to speak to a client's subconscious and can be used to reframe their negative thinking patterns. For example, someone who loves nature might respond well to a metaphor about the importance of the changing seasons.

About the Author

Nicky Peters is a creative coach, hypnotherapist and NLP practitioner with a background in graphic design. She started her career working at global publishers Penguin UK in London before moving on to designing for the fintech industry in Paris. She has since shifted from the corporate world to the wellbeing sector with a mission to inspire personal transformation and boost others' confidence to encourage a life lived more imaginatively. Currently living in Aix en Provence, France, Nicky enjoys helping individuals address their subconscious needs and develop the right mindset to lead more fulfilling lives and careers.

The Show Must Go On **33**

So Must the Process

Nicolle Nattrass

> Creativity is a wild mind and a disciplined eye.
>
> —Dorothy Parker

"The show must go on" is a common expression in the live entertainment industry. But when a pandemic hits and Broadway closes for the first time ever, creative artists like actors, playwrights, directors, designers and technical crews are left standing in the wings. With canceled contracts and creative projects on hold, creative artists faced great losses and adversity in many ways, artistically and financially.

Many of my own creative projects were also facing a state of perpetual uncertainty. I was in the process of writing a new one-woman play called *Suddenly 50* and was granted a funded residency to further its development. That residency was postponed, then canceled, not once but three times during the pandemic.

As an artist, I was accustomed to working within the parameters of uncertainty while adapting to the fluid and often nonlinear creative process. However, like the majority of artists during this time, I had never been faced with these circumstances and the new, grim reality of opportunities shutting down globally. No start date was in sight. Between adapting my own creative artist's needs and figuring out how to navigate coaching and facilitating workshops online, I leaned heavily into my support network, writing circles, fellow coaches and counselors.

A coach in my circle specialized as a business "strategy coach" and also had a previous career as an actor in New York. We ended up talking about the precarious longevity of careers as creative artists and he, in his very Rhode

DOI: 10.4324/9781003351344-33

Island/New York way, said: "Nattrass, I'm curious. I'm sure that during your theatre career, you hit many blocks and rejections along the way. What kept you going?" He offered a few coaching sessions, challenging me to focus on what I had discovered and on transforming that knowledge into a framework of action.

An avid journaler, I began writing, tuning in and reflecting on past and current creative experiences. I discovered a common denominator that I believe was the key that allowed me to complete whatever creative project I was working on. It seemed to have two components: maintaining self-care and keeping a tender heart, staying heart centered no matter the obstacles. Keeping heart centered assures that you are listening to yourself and this can lead you back to what fueled the creative work in the first place.

My colleague followed with a nudge: "Nattrass, why don't you put it in writing and send it to me." I did. The writing reflection resulted in clarifying my own creative process, defining it as a Cycle of Creative Care. It is a three-phase program, a circle that flows in either direction, depending on the needs of the client and their creative work. This creative process is nonlinear, leaving room for spontaneity, synchronicity and intuitive flow.

The Three Phases of the Cycle of Creative Care

Phase 1 - Uncover/Discover
Phase 2 - Recover/Redefine
Phase 3 - Emerge/Expand

Let me present a couple of examples.

The pandemic sent me the opportunity to begin coaching two new clients. Client #1, Melissa, was a 24-year-old actor, singer and emerging writer. She had received her first local acting award and had garnered attention from theatre professionals just as the pandemic hit. Coaching began during lockdown when she had moved back into her parents' home. She regularly suffered from anxiety, which had worsened and she was feeling lost, afraid, disassociated and unmotivated.

After the initial consultation, we established a safe, nurturing space and a reassuring routine over the online platform Zoom. When Melissa was ready, we moved into Phase 1 and spent a great deal of time exploring, uncovering and discovering not only self-care skills but also her creative goals. Those creative goals were explored during our coaching time over a year-long period. One highlight was that she became self-motivated to audition from home, which resulted in booking voice-over contracts. When theatres finally fully opened again in 2022, she auditioned and booked her first professional theatre contract.

Client #2, Christina, was a colleague and friend who became a new client. She was 50, a successful entrepreneur, writer and playwright who was venturing back into the arena of playwriting. She was also taking the risk of performing her work in a new one-woman play. Due to the level of her experience, we were beginning the Cycle of Creative Care in Phase 3. Using the language of the third phase as our compass, we seamlessly moved back and forth through the other phases. This was necessary because with the added level of performing, she was facing a greater degree of risk. The subject matter of her play was based on historic, very traumatic events, that were potentially stirring her own trauma as a creative artist as well.

The pace of progress was client led, with strong guidance and creative self-care tools provided to strengthen the foundation of confidence needed because of the level of risk involved. My coaching continued throughout the writing and rehearsal processes as well as the final performance. My overall focus became monitoring to assure that she was slowing down enough to integrate her discoveries so she would fully receive the benefits. The completion of her creative work was that her show did go on. In spite of COVID and theatres closing, she rented a theatre space and performed her new one-woman play. She adapted her performance for film with the support of a production team; the result was a captivating hybrid of both theatre and film.

The show did go on and so did the process.

 Three Tips for Creatives

1. Keep a "process journal." Let it be messy. Record, track and follow creative impulses. This can be helpful for when you get stuck or blocked as you can track back to find a piece of the puzzle or missing ingredient. For actors, I suggest keeping an audition journal to record what worked, what didn't, who you met and what you did to prepare yourself for the audition. For playwrights, focus; take time to write down a rewrite plan before you start editing your drafts. Cutting work too soon can lead to more lengthy detective work later.

2. I often say, "Pay special attention to the thoughts or feelings that you hear during the incubation or collecting stage of any creative work." If you hear yourself think, "Oh, I could never do that" or "This could never work," do not dismiss these thoughts. Instead lean in, listen, investigate.

3. Look for opportunities that give you deadlines to develop your work. If you can't find them, make them up. Deadlines can help you stay motivated. It's wise to find someone to be accountable to. For example, with my first solo play, I had an agreement with my best friend to call me every hour so that I would be less likely to procrastinate. Better yet, offer a reciprocal exchange for something they need motivation with too. It works!

 Three Tips for Coaches

1. Explore daily journal practice after client sessions. Many of the themes that emerge out of coaching sessions are often clues, prompts, or magical instances of synchronicity.

2. Strive to balance sensitivity and nurturing with holding firm to clients' goals for completion of their creative work. Stay curious and attentive to your clients' initial and ongoing access needs. Investigate what folks need for new learning or for full participation to occur. Everyone benefits from taking the extra time to find out what works best for their process, comfort and safety.

3. One of my favorite questions to ask clients is, "Do you have a sense of what the next right thing is for you? What is your best guess?" Here, I listen for clues, a kernel, a spark that emerges, listening to what is spoken as well as giving space for what is not spoken.

 ## About the Author

Nicolle Nattrass is a Certified Addiction Counselor (CAC II), playwright (PGC), professional actress (CAEA) and workshop facilitator. After a career of 20 years as a professional actor, followed by years of frontline work as an addiction counselor, she now creates journaling programs and courses that combine a therapeutic and creative approach for clients and journal keepers as well as those in other helping professions. Her first book, *Just the Two of Us (A Soft Place for Tender Hearts to Land)* was published by The Zebra Ink (2020). She is also a contributing author to the books *Transformational Journaling for Coaches & Clients: The Complete Guide to the Benefits of Personal Writing* and *The Great Book of Journaling*, co-edited by Lynda Monk and Eric Maisel. For more info, visit www.nicollenattrass.com. For links to her course and book, see www.iajw.org.

How to Stay When You Feel Like Bailing

34

Marcy Nelson-Garrison

Have you ever had a creative project where you just wanted to throw your hands in the air and give up?

There are so many ways to get thrown off track. It's like the minute you commit to creating, there is a gold embossed invitation sent to saboteur land saying, *Over here, easy prey.*

They come out in full force, saying things like "You don't have time for this"; "There are emails to respond to and research to do and invoicing"; etc. Or the super nasty "Who do you think you are? You aren't creative; this is terrible." Ugh, right?

Following creative inspiration and urges is not for the faint of heart. It requires a decision, a commitment and lots of staying power.

I'm a visual artist, but to be honest, the bulk of my creating is for my business. And I love it! Most of my clients are also creating for their businesses. My signature program is the Card Deck Master Class. Creating a card deck is an interesting project because it is an incredible vehicle for creative self-expression and it is also strategic.

The first place the saboteurs show up for my card deck class participants is to push them to leave the creative process as soon as possible and head straight for strategy. It never fails; they grab the very first idea that comes and want to run with it. My job is to keep them in the creative process long enough for a really good idea to show up. It's most often the second or third iteration that will be the standout idea.

That's one of the many places where my clients struggle with creative projects. To help them maintain creative flow, I came up with four practices that I call FLOW, STAY, LOVE and PACE. They came from my own work struggling

DOI: 10.4324/9781003351344-34

with completion. My genius coach at the time pointed out how many creative projects I had completed. She was right and we started to explore how they happened. You never know how wise you are until someone pulls it out of you. FLOW, STAY, LOVE and PACE emerged.

FLOW is all about making time to get "in the zone." That's where time seems to stand still and it's you and your project and nothing else matters. It's a state that feels good to be in.

STAY is about sticking with your project even when the inevitable saboteurs, outer critics and other bumps in the road show up.

LOVE is about remembering that this creative project isn't just another thing you have to do; it's a really cool project that you love. Sometimes we forget this!

PACE is about finding a rhythm that serves both the creator and the project. Going too fast or too slow can impact completion.

Of these four, STAY is absolutely critical to seeing a project through to completion and it covers some slippery territory.

The risk of bailing happens most often when saboteurs or our inner critics show up to tell us we aren't good enough or something equally nasty. Those messages are usually triggered by two things:

1. Discomfort in the creative process itself and/or
2. Criticism or negativity from someone else

Discomfort in the Creative Process

Discomfort is actually common in the creative process and it's not talked about much. Everyone thinks creativity is fun and play. And it is, until you bump up against what's called "creative tension." Robert Fritz is the one most associated with this concept. To simplify, you kind of see where you want to go but can't quite resolve the path to get there . . . yet.

As an artist, I've experienced this as angst or frustration. It is uncomfortable. Unfortunately, that discomfort gets misinterpreted as a sign to quit. You might hear yourself thinking, "I can't do it," and wonder if you are "just fooling yourself." Uh-oh, did you see how a sneaky saboteur just jumped on that discomfort and is now turning it into something bad?

Discomfort is not bad. It's important to remember that creative tension is normal. There is no judgment in creative tension – only discomfort and a desire to find resolution. The saboteur wants you to stop looking for resolution and bail.

When you are in the discomfort of creative tension and trying to force a resolution, it's sometimes hard to get into the flow zone. When you recognize that you are in that state, shift to another creative project for a while. There are two reasons this is helpful. Working on something else allows you to get into flow. It loosens your thinking and your attachment. There is room now for something new to show up when you return to work on the original project. Plus, science tells us there are brain chemicals associated with the flow state that linger for three to five days, so you would have that working in your favor.

Criticism or Negativity From Someone Else

The other situation that requires support to STAY is when someone criticizes your efforts or your personhood for trying something creative. Creative projects are tender in the beginning and the slightest criticism can easily deflate enthusiasm, undermine commitment and trigger your own self-judgment. STAYING is about not abandoning yourself, your ideas, or your wisdom in response to another. Feedback is ALWAYS about the person giving the feedback.

I had a powerful lesson around feedback as an artist in my very early days of exhibiting. I had two shows featuring very similar work a few months apart. Both were reviewed and the reviews were published. One reviewer said, "Why did she bother to do six of them?" (argh – a knife to the heart). The second reviewer practically wrote a love letter about the work (WOW!). Two things helped me learn from this: having an art mentor write me a note affirming my work and encouraging me to let go of the bad review *and* the second review, which was such an extreme contrast that it made it clear both reviews were about the person writing the review. Ultimately, what was most important was how I felt about the work.

This points to the importance of protecting yourself, especially early in the creative process. If someone stomps on your creative ideas and projects, call in the cavalry – get loving support.

The bottom line is your work matters. If a creative urge has called to you – hang in, stick it out, STAY the course!

 Three Tips for Creatives

Here are a few tips for STAYING no matter what . . .

1. Ask yourself, "Am I experiencing creative tension? Is there a part of my project that isn't resolving easily?" This will help you differentiate between creative tension and the sneaky, lying inner critic.

2. Be gentle with yourself. It's okay to be uncomfortable; it doesn't mean anything other than normal creative tension. Try working on a different project for a while.

3. If someone says something negative about your work and it activates your saboteur voice, pause and ask yourself some intentional questions about your work. "What do I know? What am I learning? What do I love about my project?" And get support from someone who loves you and your creativity.

 Three Tips for Coaches

For those working with creative clients, I often do a short grounding in my groups and invite reflection of the past week in terms of FLOW, STAY, LOVE and PACE.

You want to assess whether they are:

- Making time for their work
- Noticing creative tension or saboteur activity
- Forgetting why they are doing it in the first place
- Needing to adjust their creative pace

Here are three tips to help your clients STAY . . .

1. Help clients differentiate the discomfort of creative tension from an activated saboteur. These get collapsed. Teasing them apart will help your client begin to recognize the difference.

2. If your client has experienced criticism or negativity in any way around their creative process, whether real or perceived, bring buckets of tender loving care. Help your client connect to what they know about their work, what they are learning from doing the work and what they love about their creative process.

3. When the inner critic/saboteur is activated, use the tools you know already. Don't be surprised when perfectionism, impatience and judgment show up. This simple message from a friend of mine is helpful: "Don't stomp on the baby shoots just because they aren't full-grown plants yet."

The creative process, whether the end result is a masterpiece or not, is powerful, healing, expanding and tender. Bring lots of love to it.

About the Author

Marcy Nelson-Garrison, MA, CPCC, is a product coach and visual artist. She founded the Coaching Toys online store, which features creative tools for workshops, retreats, team building and client work. Marcy loves introducing coaches to creative processes that enhance their work with clients. Clients hire Marcy when they are ready to create powerful products and programs that reflect who they are, make a difference and make money. Marcy is the creator of the popular Card Deck Master Class and The Product Lab. Learn more at www.pinkparadigm.com.

Neuronal Energy Shot　**35**

Using Guided Imagery to Activate Performance Energy

Denise Wonnerth

Some clients struggle to plan their creative work; others get lost somewhere during the process. Then there are clients who completely break down and feel paralyzed inches before the finish line. This chapter presents some ideas on working with guided imagery to provide and nurture artists with the energy boost, so sorely needed, that finishing their creative process will provide.

Even though it focuses on completing creative work, the tool itself can be used throughout your creative work. You can build your personal safe place, plan your whole creative process by combining guided imagery with timelines, or visit a source of inspiration and energy, whenever you require it.

Sarah and Her Undernourished Diminishing Performance Energy

A new coaching client showed up – let's call her Sarah – telling me that she felt completely stressed and burned out. By the time she came for coaching, she was working on her second novel – her award-winning debut had been published years ago.

Sarah had started her creative work with enthusiasm and confidence. She handled the smaller ups and downs at the beginning and now, almost finished, she had just stopped. She was demoralized and had no idea what had happened to her dream.

DOI: 10.4324/9781003351344-35

She thought she knew everything about the challenges creatives faced because she'd already written and published a novel. But she was proven wrong. What she didn't have in mind was that every creative process comes with its very own creative challenges. The challenges she faced years ago had nothing in common with those she was facing right now.

Sarah was losing contact with herself and her project. A second novel felt like a heavy burden. Friends and relatives were asking her about the book. Her agent got impatient and was prodding her to finish it. A feeling of emptiness and insecurity took over inside her. She'd spent so much time on her work and now it all felt like a failure.

She lost her drive and didn't even know what she was doing it for. Her vision faded, her energy drained out and her self-esteem vanished. With permission to take over, her doubts had a green light. In no time, they gained the upper hand over her thoughts and feelings. Convinced that her award-winning debut was just a bit of luck, she talked herself into a spiral of negativity, fueled by dubious advice from people who were either sitting in the same boat or who meant well but were ultimately not really being supportive.

Sarah was unable to appreciate her first publication, the hard work that was rewarded and praised and she felt stuck. She explained:

> Nobody would have cared about my first novel if the market had offered more interesting books. I can't write a single line. I'm a living proof of failure. How can I consider myself being a writer? That's so pathetic. By publishing a second work, I will just out myself as a lousy impostor. And everyone will know it. Critics are going to tear me and my work to pieces. Everyone says that the second book is far harder than the first one. Expectations are higher; readers are more critical. I guess I'm just not made of writers' material. Giving up is the only option left.

During our coaching together, we used guided imagery several times with the goal of getting her self-esteem back on track. She needed to get rid of, or at least decrease, her negativity and realize that she was a talented writer. As a result of doing this, her sense of self-efficacy returned and she found it easier to be more positive. The visualizations allowed her to appreciate her achievements and everything she had accomplished so far. This helped her feel more confident again.

Finally, visualizing her completed creative project through guided imagery provided her with the performance energy she needed to cross the finish line and get her novel done.

Guided Imagery

Guided imagery is essentially a relaxation technique that comes with many benefits. Regular use of guided imagery has a structure-forming effect on our brain and helps reduce anxiety, sharpen concentration and increase creativity. It's a method for managing stress by visualizing positive and peaceful settings, one that we can also use to boost our performance energy and nurture our creative soul with positive vibes and motivation.

Visualize Your Success

"What we think, we become." We all know the Buddha's quote and yet we barely consider it; rather, we indulge ourselves in negative thoughts. Sarah's struggle is a common phenomenon in a creative's world. The nearer the work's completion, the tenser we get on the inside. Instead of focusing on ourselves and our feelings, we are suddenly focused more on outside worries and fears. We wonder if people will like our creative work, what critics might say about it, whether it will be as good as the creations of others. The solution? Stop wondering and stop comparing!

If we start caring more about the external factors at the completion stage of our creative process, we'll hardly finish. All those fears and doubts will drain us. So, instead of negative thinking that holds us down, why not think positive thoughts, imagining our success, nurturing our creative soul with love and devotion?

What You Need to Get Started With Guided Imagery

Guided imagery can be done anytime and anywhere. Used as a relaxation technique, it doesn't require any special equipment or knowledge. In general, you just need a quiet spot and a comfortable/convenient place to sit or lie down.

If you don't use it as a relaxation technique but as a method to visualize completing or planning projects, I recommend working with another person. A coach or a good friend can help you dig deeper and get more insights and benefits out of it.

Sit in a quiet and safe place and relax. Take a few calming breaths. Begin to think about your work. Close your eyes and imagine that you just completed your creative project. Think of all the details linked to that idea. Try answering the following questions in the most precise way possible:

- Sights: What do you see? Where are you and what is surrounding you? Any dominating colors? People? Landscape? A gallery or a bookstore?
- Sounds: What do you hear? Any kind of melody, voices, or sounds? A cheering crowd? Birds? Water? Music? Silence?
- Tactile feelings: What feelings and sensations are you aware of? What does completing your creative work feel like? Where can you locate those emotions, feelings and sensations within your body?
- Smells: What do you smell? How does it smell? Does the smell ring a bell, reminding you of anything familiar?
- Tastes: Can you taste something? What do you taste? How does it taste?

Sarah began moving nervously while visualizing the completion of her project, telling me all the details. She found herself in a crowded but bright room. It took a while until she figured out that she was at a book reading. People were whispering, sometimes sighing. Her heartbeat quickened and she started sweating. She saw her words written on the pages of her book. Turning pages, she felt the paper's texture under her fingertips. There was that typical smell of a new book and its ink. It was a good feeling. She knew it. It reminded her of all the situations in her life that she had successfully managed even if they frightened her. Her whole posture changed. She was fully energized and stimulated. She had a smile all over her face.

We used hypnotic anchoring to establish a trigger for her emotional state to make sure she could easily get back and access that motivating and vitalizing feeling. The more you get into your visualization, the more energy you can extract and bring to your creative performance and completion. The resonating perception is bound to provoke vivid sensations so you're chomping at the bit to complete your work, just as Sarah was.

Just be sure to remember that visualizations do not replace actions! No picture, no novel and no song is created and realized in your mind. Your mind is not the spot where action takes place. Visualizing doesn't substitute for the hard work that you will have to face, but positive thoughts and neuronal energy make hard work easier.

Three Tips for Creatives

1. You are greater than the sum of your creative products. Remember, a creative life, or rather a creative's life, is a mosaic of countless creative processes. The single pieces of a creation might be imperfect, but once you've seen the entire picture, you're overwhelmed by its complexity and perfection. Some projects might fail, while others will blaze. Nevertheless, as creatives, we need all of them to become better. So go ahead and fail forward.

2. Nurture your creative soul. Provide yourself with curiosity, impartiality and the irrepressible joy of experimentation. Get in touch with your needs regularly. Ask yourself, "What does my creative soul require for charging my batteries and where can I get that?"

3. Build your own community. Yes, you are responsible for your creative work and the creative process. You are the one in charge of building and establishing a supporting environment for yourself. But being responsible is not the equivalent of being alone! Build a community with supporters who encourage one another and whose feedback is of real use to you to help keep you going and to provide resources.

 Three Tips for Coaches

1. Be curious and go for more. Whatever your clients are describing, dig deeper and ask for more details, more sensations. Escort your clients with the curiosity and the eyes of a child.

2. Pay attention to the coherence of statements and body language. Our bodies reveals so much more information than words ever will. If you notice any kind of dissonance, you might say something like "You just told me how great completing your painting would feel, but you mentioned there has been that lump in your throat and I just wondered if there's anything you're worried about?"

3. Offer without imposing. Some clients lack the words to describe feelings, situations, or even their visualizations. Offer metaphors or suggest other adjectives but do not insist that your client accept them.

About the Author

Denise Wonnerth is a systemic consultant and creativity coach. She holds a diploma in adult education and is also certified in working with gifted clients. Denise has ten years of teaching and coaching experience and, as a writing enthusiast, has to deal with all the challenges of the creative process herself. Learn more at www.sichtveksel.com.

Timely Completing Using Your Existential Intelligence

36

Eric Maisel

You will find it easier to complete your works of art if you hold that completing them matters to you. That is, you need a certain existential decisiveness to combat all the reasons for not completing.

But where does this existential decisiveness come from and how can you cultivate more of it? To answer this important question, we need to look at a subject that may be unfamiliar to you: the idea of existential intelligence. Please join me as we explore this quite underexplored subject.

For the past hundred years, people have been thought of – and thought of themselves – as falling somewhere along a continuum of intelligence that ran from incredibly high to above average to average to below average. It was never clear "how much" intelligence any of these stops along the continuum represented, so it was quite impossible to say whether a person of average intelligence had "enough" intelligence for a particular task, whether that task was learning theoretical physics or voting in an election. It was simply taken for granted that average intelligence – the intelligence manifested by most people – was "good enough" to handle the ordinary tasks of living. And if it wasn't – well, what was the individual, society, or species to do about that shortfall?

Since so much about the concept of intelligence remained unexamined and unclear, it became increasingly easy to argue that intelligence tests did little more than measure whatever the creator of the test happened to be in the mood to measure. Such tests apparently told us very little about "real intelligence," "raw intelligence," or "natural intelligence." Since no other instruments were available to measure "real," "raw," or "natural" intelligence,

DOI: 10.4324/9781003351344-36

a new way of looking at intelligence was bound to emerge. So we began to hear about a new fish in the sea: "multiple intelligences."

Howard Gardner, the originator of this way of conceptualizing intelligence, argued that human beings possessed not a single unitary intelligence but several distinct intelligences. He named seven and then added an eighth: linguistic intelligence ("word smart, as in a poet"); logical-mathematical intelligence ("number/reasoning smart, as in a scientist"); spatial intelligence ("picture smart, as in a sculptor or airplane pilot"); bodily-kinesthetic intelligence ("body smart, as in an athlete or dancer"); musical intelligence ("music smart, as in a composer"); interpersonal intelligence ("people smart, as in a salesman or teacher"); intrapersonal intelligence ("self-smart, exhibited by individuals with accurate views of themselves"); and, later, naturalist intelligence ("nature smart, as in a naturalist").

Because his scheme served many agendas, it caught on quickly. When Daniel Goleman proposed another intelligence, emotional intelligence, it likewise found a large, sympathetic audience. Anyone good at networking but bad at chemistry could now think of himself as "just as intelligent" as that boy in high school chemistry class who memorized the periodic table at a glance. Who wouldn't embrace the idea that whatever you happened to be good at made you something of a genius?

At the end of the day, however, we were still left with a large hole in the middle of the intelligence discussion. Even a moment's thought forced one to realize just how many disparate ideas – how many apples, oranges and pears – were being squashed together into the intelligence package: natural differences, cultural differences, experiential differences, attitudinal differences, motivational differences and so on. More important, every formulation of intelligence, whether of the unitary or the multiple sort, failed to address the following vital question: what intelligence or aspect of intelligence allowed you to comprehend what anything *meant*?

No one tackled the central question of what intelligence or aspect of intelligence allowed a person to comprehend what anything meant. Let's do that right now and embrace the idea of existential intelligence, an intelligence that must exist if our felt sense of meaning exists. Existential intelligence is the intelligence that concerns itself with what things mean. It is that part of our nature that steps back, slips on a wide-angle lens and appraises in the realm of meaning. It is our first, primary and most important intelligence because it and only it, allows us to know what to do with our other intelligences. We may be capable in any number of ways, but we are just a bundle of capabilities until we apply our existential intelligence. All the other intelligences are capabilities, but existential intelligence is the coordinating intelligence, the intelligence that all the other intelligences serve.

Existential intelligence can be construed as the capacity for conceptualizing deeper or larger questions about human existence, such as the meaning of life, why we are born, why we die, what consciousness is and how we got here. It is all that, but it is also much more. It is the intelligence we use to appraise the meaning of our life minute by minute. It is existential intelligence that permits us to think through whether we should fight in a war or protest a war, renew our efforts to live or take our life, embrace our culture or rebel against it. Anything that we intend to do thoughtfully in the realm of values requires the application of our existential intelligence.

None of the other intelligences help us know how we should construct meaning in our life. That we are fluent with words, fit for the Royal Ballet, or can out-sketch Picasso doesn't help us know what we should do with that capability – or why we should use it at all. Existential intelligence is the only human faculty that permits a person to think in the domain of meaning, to make decisions about meaning and to actively construct meaning. It is time we acknowledged its central role in human affairs and recognized how the personal application of existential intelligence can lead to amazing triumphs in the realm of meaning.

For a creative person, countless questions arise in the realm of meaning, questions like the following:

- Why should I bother to paint?
- Why should I paint this and not that?
- Why should I paint this subject matter when that subject matters sells better?
- Why should I paint when, if I'm lucky enough to sell a painting, it will merely end up hanging in a dentist's office?
- Why should I paint when I could contribute more by simply being of service?
- Why should I bother completing my current painting?

Existential intelligence is a significant force in your life – the most significant, really – because, while it is a demanding intelligence, a driving intelligence and a pestering intelligence, it is also essential for guidance. It might be nice to surgically remove this pesky part of our inheritance; then we could simply do what others told us to do or what felt good to do. But how would we go about removing that part of our makeup? And would we really want to remove it, thereby dooming ourselves to slavery and conventionality?

Existential intelligence is indeed pesky, but it also provides real direction and the best answers. It demands not only that you pick a direction but also that you justify your pick smartly and convincingly. It likewise helps you identify that direction and make sense of your choices. This discussion may have brought an old-fashioned word to mind: the word *conscience*. Existential intelligence is to meaning what conscience is to morals: both pester but also provide guidance.

It is actually fortunate that we have existential intelligence and a conscience because they and the institutions that spring from them, keep civilization civil, enlightened and humane.

It is also an unfortunate thing, as neither existential intelligence nor conscience ever sleeps and both are hard to satisfy. You come up with what feels like a meaningful reason to paint images of radishes and your existential intelligence pipes up with, "Yes, well, I get that, but looked at from another point of view, I'm not sure you're justified. And what if we look at the matter from this other angle? And this other angle?" Existential intelligence, like conscience, may save the species, but it surely badgers the individual.

It is your existential intelligence that causes you to have no doubts about your path on Monday and serious doubts on Tuesday. You feel comfortable with your imagery choices in January and are bored with them in February. You are fine with the machinations of the marketplace in the morning and have to shake your head at them in the evening. Subjective meaning shifts according to our shifting appraisal of what is right, proper and defensible to do and according to our sense of the value of our actions and intentions. All this turbulence is the fruit of our existential intelligence at work.

Is this significant pressure in the area of meaning a positive or a negative force in an artist's life? Insofar as it forces us to try to do our best and be our best and helps us actively make meaning, discern our path and our reasons for choosing it and contribute to the betterment of our species and our world, existential intelligence is a positive. Insofar as it badgers us about our choices, heaps mile-high doubts on our meaning constructions and looks at our every choice from so many angles as to give us a migraine, it is a powerful emotional negative. So what is it on balance?

That depends in large measure on the relationship you craft with your existential intelligence. If you can enter into a smart, compassionate dialogue with yourself about how you intend to handle meaning crises and real-world challenges and if you can skillfully parlay your natural existential savvy into periodic moments of existential joy, your existential intelligence will prove a blessing. If, on the other hand, you forego such conversations, you are likely to end up feeling battered in the realm of meaning – and one natural consequence of that battering is that you will find yourself less likely to complete your creative projects.

Your existential intelligence becomes a positive when you enlist it in the service of passionately making meaning. This smart use of your existential intelligence is a four-step process, beginning with the decision to matter. First, you decide that you will live a principled, creative, active life in support of your cherished ideals; that you will manifest your potential; that you will do good work – that, in short, you will make your life matter, on your own terms and at least to you. You do not presume that your life matters on a cosmic scale or that your efforts will move mountains. Rather, you embrace the idea of authenticity and proclaim that you intend to live an authentic life.

Second, having decided that you intend to matter, you announce the following: "Irrespective of whether the universe is meaningful or meaningless, irrespective of whether my odds of succeeding are long or short, irrespective of everything at the existential level and at the practical level, I am going to intentionally make meaning." You decide to matter and then you announce that you intend to make sufficient meaning in and for your life. You embrace the following core idea: there is no meaning "out there" to locate; there are only our subjective sense of meaning and our efforts at making and maintaining meaning.

Third, ask yourself the question, "Well, then, what exactly are my life purposes? If I'm going to actively make meaning in accordance with my life purposes, I had better know them, articulate them, memorize them and make sure that I really believe in them. So what are they?" That is, you need to identify your real reasons for living and the role or roles you intend to play in life. Your life purposes may be to fight against injustice, to live a life better than your baser instincts, to make beautiful things, to do good deeds and so on. These are the sorts of life purposes that are rich enough and big enough to count.

Fourth, you need to tackle all this with passion and energy. Remember that you are *passionately* making meaning. It might seem to go without saying that a person would naturally be passionate about something as central and vital to their life as their own life purposes. However, we know this isn't true. Few people live their lives passionately. Most people go through the motions in life, burdened by their tasks, their everyday work, their responsibilities and their own personality. They live closer to depression than ecstasy, often in a perpetual meaning crisis. Indeed, most people need convincing that it makes sense to be passionate about anything.

Let me repeat these four steps:

1. You decide to matter.
2. You accept that you must make meaning.
3. You identify your life purposes and articulate a life purpose statement.
4. You passionately act to fulfill your life purposes.

The phrase that I'm using to encompass these four ideas is *passionately making meaning*. When, employing your existential intelligence, you arrive at these conclusions, you will have acquired a much more solid existential footing and will find it much easier to complete your creative projects.

At the heart of a creative act like painting, sculpting, screenwriting, song-writing, or any other creative act is the effort to make meaning (and not just beautiful objects or money). We are happy if we make objects we like and if we make money, but what we are really after as we create is the experience of making our life feel meaningful. Completing our creative projects makes our life feel more meaningful. *That's* why we finish things: for the sake of that special psychological feeling.

 Three Tips for Creatives

1. How would you describe *existential intelligence* in your own words?
2. Does the phrase make sense to you? If so, in what ways?
3. How might you make better use of your existential intelligence when it comes to completing your creative projects?

 Three Tips for Coaches

1. The phrase *existential intelligence* may not be part of your vocabulary and you may have no experience in using it. How might you chat with clients about the ideas discussed in this chapter, using your own language?

2. Think about the paradigm shift from "the purpose of life" to the idea of "multiple life purposes." Does that resonate with you? If it does, how might you communicate that idea in session?
3. What are your thoughts about the connection between existential issues and completing creative work?

 ## About the Author

Eric Maisel is the author of 50+ books. His recent books include *Why Smart Teens Hurt, Redesign Your Mind* and *The Power of Daily Practice.* Among his other books are *Coaching the Artist Within, Fearless Creating, Rethinking Depression* and *The Van Gogh Blues.* Dr. Maisel writes the *Rethinking Mental Health* blog for *Psychology Today,* with 3,000,000+ views and is the creator and lead editor for the Ethics International Press Critical Psychology and Critical Series. A retired family therapist and active creativity coach, Dr. Maisel's forthcoming books include *The Coach's Way* (New World Library) and *Deconstructing ADHD* (Ethics International Press). Dr. Maisel provides workshops, webinars and keynotes nationally and internationally; trains creativity coaches; and facilitates support groups for writers. You can visit him at www.ericmaisel.com and contact him at ericmaisel@hotmail.com.

Encouraging Motivation During the Final Stages

37

Aneesah Wilhelmstätter

Are you running out of steam and is completion feeling like a drag? Or perhaps your initial "high" has fallen flat? Maybe it's that the pressure has built up into a storm of agitation? Whether you are a writer, a painter, a performer, or some other creative professional, you're not alone. What's important now is how to reignite your creative spark and connect to the wellspring within to deliver on your great work.

Gabriel, a top Michelin Star chef, came to me with this kind of frustrated motivation. Not managing to bridge the gap to deliver on his cookbook, he was feeling constantly on edge. While his unwholesome motivational strategies of will power, harsh self-criticism, fear and booze – lots of it – had gotten him his first and subsequent stars, they were no longer serving him. While this master chef *knew* in a rational way the importance of bringing his book project to completion, it was not translating into a *visceral* experience. He was primed for some creative change.

Another client, Elizabeth, one year from retiring from her IT job, came to me with a similar struggle. Whenever she thought of setting up her photography website to market her offerings, her positive drive took a downward dive, often with severe migraine headaches the only thing to show for it. Confident about her photography abilities and tech savvy and with an amazing portfolio on her hard drive, this particular type of drive issue was getting the better of her.

These are only two of the many stories of perfectly capable creatives, struggling needlessly to stay motivated during the final stages of their projects. Before getting on with their project, they typically want to figure out

DOI: 10.4324/9781003351344-37

"How come this is so?" As valid a line of inquiry as this is, to begin there in our work together would amount to another destructive, distracting strategy.

Denial, the defensive attempt to avoid looking at how I get in my own way, is something I, too, know all too well. How often have I believed that the thing to do was to deny unpleasant experiences, such as the difficult thoughts and emotions around completion and just do it? Denial is the defense mechanism, the reactivity that leads us all to making destructive decisions, with their consequent destructive, if not dangerous outcomes.

I have learned that, to give my clients true value, I needed to start our sessions as a mindfulness coach. Yes, I meet them where they're at, with the questions they are wrestling with: what to do and what not to do. I also invite them to a new kind of dance – the tantalizing tango between "being" and "doing." Mindfully present myself, I give my clients the gift of mindful presence. By teaching them the "how" of cultivating present-moment awareness, they learn to bring themselves to a state of "being" to support their important do-it-now goals.

STOP and SIT is a humble and simple operating system I've designed to help my clients encourage the necessary motivation to complete their victory lap – with calm strength, ease and joy. This method takes direct aim at the root cause of our struggles with motivation, thus liberating us from our dusty denial coveralls to create lasting positive change.

With this in mind, whatever is or isn't happening in our world at the moment, we start with STOP. STOP (surrender, slow it down, pause and halt) is the first of this operating system's four simple steps. And there's no denying that this is not easy. Probably the hardest step of all is to stop doing and to stop distracting ourselves as a way to flee unpleasant experiences. When we are feeling hijacked by our past habits, including distracting ourselves from being present to our present-moment experiences, stopping is the thing to do. And, from this new spacious awareness, we make the next steps possible.

This is where SIT comes in. And no, "SIT" doesn't mean you are being ordered to sit down and just do it. Rather, it is an invitation to take a seat at the table. The *S* in the acronym SIT is for *self-direct*. What it takes to develop this primary mental fitness muscle, Shirzad Chamine tells us in his book *Positive Intelligence*, is the regular application of ten-second "reps" of focused attention. What you are doing for each ten-second self-leadership rep is, in effect, calming your survival brain to tip into the green zone – and it's good to be home.

Gabriel, our accomplished chef, stopped to practice listening to the sounds around him with "exquisite" attention. Elizabeth, our photographer, focused on her breathing without trying to change it. Alternatively, she offered herself some much-needed self-friendliness by mentally repeating phrases like "May I be joyful" and "May I be well." Surfing the waves of my sensory experience while mentally noting "pleasant," "unpleasant," or "neutral" to describe my changing experiences of sounds and other sensations is how I choose to "be with" myself and center.

Sometimes, simply stopping to sit with our experience for ten seconds can give us all the freedom we need to move onto doing what needs to be done. In the long run, deliberately practicing introducing a fresh perspective makes for a more robust motivational experience. This is where the *I* in SIT, which stands for *introduction*, serves us well. Introducing interest, self-inquiry and a fresh perspective intercepts old patterns to create new possibilities.

Simply asking myself, "What do I get from this?" creates a kind of disenchantment with destructive and costly coping strategies. Then, less resistant and more open, I can introduce a more creative perspective. Asking herself this question when her headaches came on helped Elizabeth widen her window of tolerance for discomfort. She started to notice that her habit of resisting her feelings created stress and the consequent migraines. For Gabriel, becoming a positive inquirer by asking the unfinished question, "Wouldn't it be wonderful . . .?" helped him break his harsh and hostile self-talk spell.

The *T* in SIT is for *transformation*. We can mindfully engage the third factor of this operating system to transform our destructive habits, like self-doubt and the drive for distraction, into something constructive. To facilitate this creative change of encouraging positive motivation, I've adapted the following exercise from Rick Hanson's book *Hardwiring Happiness*. First, you identify the subtasks that it would serve you to "want." Then you continue by making a list of the benefits in becoming more naturally motivated to complete these subtasks. Also include the intrinsic benefits – perhaps around the skills you are building – such as interpersonal skills, setting healthy boundaries, recognizing your worth and how this will benefit you, etc. Repeat this mindfulness practice while working on the subtask and again at the end of the working session.

While the STOP and SIT operating system helps my clients, including Gabriel and Elizabeth, joyfully move through the final stages of their projects, thereby increasing the likelihood of worldly success, none of us can control how our work is received. However, through mindfulness and focusing on the benefits of subjectively unpleasant tasks, we all get better at savoring the success of authentic completion and can still feel successful no matter what the objective outcome.

Three Tips for Creatives

The following tips will help enrich and deepen your practice by introducing a sense of ritual and ceremony.

1. Hone your focus and supercharge your motivation with power words. Do this around those pesky subtasks by reading out loud from your list of "benefits of completion."
2. Power up your creative space with words, images and icons of inspiration. Connect especially with things of sentimental value that inspire a positive experience.
3. Choose and regularly activate an embodied experience of calm strength and positive motivation. Energizing yourself with a power move, pose, or posture can support your intentions to complete your work.

 ### Three Tips for Coaches

The following tips for coaches relate to installing a daily practice.

1. Consistently hold a supportive space for your clients to reflect on the benefits of wanting new things and to share their STOP and SIT joys and challenges.
2. Regularly adopting an attitude of playful experimentation helps your clients grow in a joyous and spontaneous way.
3. Highlighting an overarching theme such as Creatively Change Your Mind adds value and makes it easy and fun for clients to apply this mindfulness technique elsewhere: for example, to creatively changing their mind about something that bothers them about another person.

About the Author

Aneesah Wilhelmstätter is a creativity and creative change coach as well as a self-taught artist who has exhibited and sold her work at prime venues like the KunstRAI in Amsterdam in 2001. As a writer, her work can be found in *Psychology Today, Thrive Global, The Creativity Workbook for Coaches and Creatives* (2020) and *Transformational Journaling for Coaches, Therapists and Clients* (2021). She is a practice leader on Integral Life and a licensed positive neuroplasticity training teacher. Her website is https://creativechange coaching.wordpress.com/.

Creative Mental Fitness

38

Nefeli Soteriou

To succeed in anything, you need to plan for it and apply effective strategies. If you want a fit body, then you need to exercise, eat nutritional foods, sleep well and trust in the process. You can't rush to fitness; if you try, you'll get injured. As you build leaner muscle, you feel and look great! In a similar manner, to complete your work of genius, you must learn to develop a mentally fit mind. By establishing a daily creative practice, you grow mental fitness muscles over time. The results of a fit mind are obvious; you get your animation pilot ready for submission, your time-based installation is photographed, your feature-length film goes out for distribution, your set of new images is out to the printer!

The majority of us know what we need to do, yet we are challenged to do it. Eating out, for example, is more convenient than bothering to cook healthy meals at home. Avoiding work on your artistic creation or trusting "What's the point?" thinking prolongs getting your masterpiece done.

One of the ways that I work with clients is to help them clarify their desires and teach them to think positively about themselves and their own capabilities to overcome difficulties. In the process, we work through examining false belief systems and behavioral and thinking patterns while learning essential life foundational principles.

Taking Responsibility

By applying cognitive-behavioral therapy techniques, I help clients start noticing the thoughts that they have. Most of the time, these thoughts are looped,

DOI: 10.4324/9781003351344-38

recycled patterns of perception. Inevitably, they affect the client's thinking, feeling and ability to regulate their actions.

"The first boundary to set for you is with you. This entails getting a grip on you and your own mind," I frequently explain. Help your clients become directive managers of their freely roaming minds. "But of course," you may say, "my clients are already very responsible." Well, I talk about the responsibility we all have as individuals to create the results we want to see in our lives and to take the road with personal meaning. Creating meaning is about causing something to appear that you want to come into being, something that would not naturally evolve or that is not made by ordinary processes.

For example, think of a seed planted in fertile ground. Even though it will most likely grow to become a tall plant, the seed still needs to be watered and nourished and the weeds to be removed frequently. You are the horticulture expert in your client's life. First, guide them to envision the end result. The in-between steps you will handle together as your partnership unfolds. Last, acting as their backbone support, see them through it. There is nothing your client can't be or do once they take responsibility for it. And that's what you can bring to the table for them, an emphasis on individual responsibility.

Keeping Promises

Most of us are subject to external influences: television, politics, society, school, culture, family. We can't really stop these. We can acknowledge that, while we will be influenced all the time, we are in control of our own actions, thoughts and feelings. By knowing that we are the authority, we can accept or reject information and the invitations offered by others. We can prioritize getting our creative work done. That's the way to live up to one's vow to complete projects.

Remind clients to celebrate their small wins toward attaining their goals. It is a self-loving act to stand back and keep things in balance. Having a good time is as important as fulfilling one's promises.

Your words have power. Your verbal communication during a coaching session reinforces your clients' transformation. I strive to use rich short sentences with visual connotations. "Stick to your vision like honey" is one of my favorite metaphors. Based on the same empowering premise, I will offer a tailored journaling prompt. You can suggest, for example, that your clients storyboard their honey-like vision or make a video of it.

Cultivating Courage

Help clients face life with courage and take life's many issues as natural occurrences. I have found that clients are more equipped to solve problems when they recognize them as an integral part of life. Provide systems that help them thrive under pressure. For example, preplanning a week's meals on a Sunday is an effective system for someone who wants to lose weight. A predesigned visual you send in between calls can uplift your client and inspire them toward their new art piece. Ask them to post these reminders in visible places. Better yet, ask them to come up with their own idea of a personal motivational visual poster. This activity can be so much fun!

Be pragmatic and compassionate as sickness and hardship are real, emotional loss is painful and the steps toward healing can be exhausting. As clients develop mental strength to resist opposition, danger, or hardship, they can begin to manifest an unyielding will in the face of danger or extreme difficulty. Sometimes being courageous means upgrading one's personality. That way, clients handle life challenges with a new perspective.

Take Mira. Mira is an accomplished props producer for theatre and television. Although she had effective systems in place, in just one day, they flew out the window at a social gathering. It was something her aunt said, a remark about her career. Fear and doubt crept in; a "What if this won't work?" thought suddenly blocked her. "My brain and body are switched off," Mira explained. "I am feeling I have no energy and can barely manage day to day tasks."

Even world-renowned professional athletes have bad days. They don't beat the drum and confess how hard it is; rather, they quickly do what they must to get back on track. After our call together, Mira sent an email: "I already feel better. I am who I am and I enjoy where I am in my profession."

 Three Tips for Creatives

1. Ask for help. Know that you are not alone. At any given moment, you can reach out for advice. You can find a suitable coaching match by exploring your options. Trust in your evaluation when a coaching partnership is not a good match. When you find the right fit, it will be magical!

2. This is, I believe. Very few things are impossible in life. I want you to have clarity in your belief system that whatever you want to achieve is always available to you. First, you need to aim to become more

honest with yourself when you don't want to do something, like completing a showpiece. The following activity will help you receive insights, renew your enthusiasm and, get work done.

Part A: Schedule some time in a private, comfortable place. Choose one of the following prompts to respond to: "I don't have the time . . .," "I am too old . . .," "I am not ready . . .," "The timing is not right . . .," etc. If another prompt is more suitable to your situation, use that one instead. You put down your thoughts in the form of automatic writing. You open up without thinking about grammar or punctuation. One page or three paragraphs are sufficient.

Part B: Come up with an affirmative response. Your prompt is "I am quickly and decisively getting there." For example," I am quickly and decisively finishing casting my protagonist this week." Last, transfer your response onto a fresh page. Write it down ten times. Post the page where you can see it.

3. A thick shield. Sit in a comfortable position in a quiet, private space. Your palms comfortably rest on your legs; your feet are grounded. Close your eyes. Inhale and exhale slowly for a few minutes, aiming to completely relax. As you continue relaxing more and more deeply, I would like you to imagine a beam of pure white light from the sky entering your crown chakra. It is a special kind of light with extraordinary shielding properties!

    As the white light gradually fills your body through your head, it goes all the way down to your feet, warming your feet, relaxing your feet, soothing your feet and grounding you as it exits to the depths of the earth. You are one with the earth and unbeatable. Feel the bright light through your eyes, relaxing your nose, soothing your ears, lips and cheeks.

    This warm light is now expanding through your neck and shoulders, chest, arms and palms, all the way to your fingertips. You are feeling stronger and stronger as this vibrant white light travels to your abdominal and pelvic area. It is relaxing your hips completely and flows down to your knees and toes. You are now fully covered by the clear light; it is translucent and carries no weight.

    Confidently now, see it expand outside you for about an inch all around you. Light as a feather, the white light shield goes anywhere you take it. You are protected. Any potential harm directed toward you is bouncing off you and away from you. Your shield is stronger than steel and you are untouchable. This visualization can protect you energetically: create it and then take a little time, on the order of ten minutes, before resuming your activities.

Three Tips for Coaches

1. Encourage your clients to take personal responsibility.
2. Help your clients notice and change their self-talk.
3. Discuss with your clients the ways that they can manifest and increase their courage.

 About the Author

Nefeli Soteriou produces independent films and helps time-based artists trust their inspirations and pursue work and a lifestyle that really fascinates them. Connect with Nefeli at www.nefelisoteriou.com.

Sylvia and Her One Thing

39

Pragati Chaudhry

Sylvia loved life and really enjoyed waking up to her art. She found her life's purpose in painting and lived it with enthusiasm. She was never worried about ideas – they came like the rain! Her work was sought after; every brushstroke she made earned her money.

After years of practice and dedication, Sylvia was in a place she wanted herself to be. She enjoyed grinding pigments and painting with them and her enthusiastic energy came through in her art pieces. She sold paintings even before they were completed. There were many collectors who expressed interest in her work, so many that it seemed that the paintings she might make in the next ten years were already spoken for.

"It's amazing to know that every brushstroke has the love that I'm trying to convey. I really enjoy the smell of paint and most of all, I love to have my coffee while looking at my painting in progress and thinking about what to do next," said Sylvia to me in our first meeting.

She went on to say, "But, in the quietness of my studio and even amongst the loveliness of all the colors, I miss belonging to a family and knowing that there is someone who can look after me and I can look after." It was important for her to have a relationship now that she was established in her career.

And, by her own admission, it was as if the moment she decided this, the universe provided for her. She started expanding her circle and meeting more and more people and just seeing where life would take her. When she came across her soulmate, she knew it. She knew what she was missing and said yes! She had the wedding of her dreams and they moved into a new house with space for her studio. She had always dreamed of a house overlooking a lake, with pristine colors and just the right light that would help her paint.

DOI: 10.4324/9781003351344-39

It was all good until the time came for her to complete the series for her next exhibition. She had completed all but the showstopper painting and was supposed to submit it to the gallery that represented her. According to her contract, she was to produce an exhibit every fall. She was now in that place where all the thinking was complete and she had to start creating that last painting. Over the next several weeks, Sylvia found herself in the place where she just could not complete it. She was unable to connect with her work, even in her lovely space – her dream studio.

As we worked together, I noticed the happiness in her voice when she talked about her married life. It was hard to tell that there was something in the way of her creative expression, her artwork and the commitment to create and complete her yearly show with this gallery. What could be going on?

"I need to submit my painting and it's so strange. I seem to have a creative block. I cannot visualize my creation anymore."

She was taking the generic steps of overcoming a "creative block," but was not able to be her creative self in her new studio. In our sessions, I began to wonder if there was "one thing" locking her up, one particular thing. Often, there is exactly one thing standing in the way of our getting our creative work done. Until we identify and handle that one thing, we are unlikely to get our work finished. Sylvia and I started our journey of identifying that "one thing" – and what to do to deal with it – so that she could bring her final big canvas into the gallery.

I asked her what this final canvas would look like. She said, "It would feel like freedom: pursuing my love, doing what I'm passionate about." I asked her how she could get there. She said, "I need to find my ease with my creative process again." "How?" I asked. What, I wondered, did she need to do first? Her answer became her action steps: 1) create color studies and 2) make sketches.

In the next session, it was exhilarating to see that Sylvia had followed her action steps, trying to establish a balance between her deadline and rekindling her creative expression, after the major life changes of marriage and moving into a new house and studio. "It is so nice to find myself creating, even though it was outside the studio, at the beach and the cafe!"

Things were going well and she was ready to work on the big canvas, the exhibit's showstopper. But when it came to facing it, she found herself experiencing panic. "I feel like this canvas and this exhibition aren't meant to be. When I am working on this piece, I feel like I am jeopardizing something!"

Sylvia didn't have a creative block because she was able to sketch and paint outside her house, nor was she afraid of failure. But there were clearly some old gremlins coming up that made her insecure. We talked about the many life transitions she had recently undergone.

"They were all joyful," she said. But something was disorienting her and causing a loss of stability. It was emotional. I suggested an exercise that I do frequently. I asked her to bring her attention to her final canvas and visualize herself as if she was completing it in her studio. I asked her to then name what voices came up. The exercise is called "two voices within."

She named one voice "artist" and the other voice "lonely." Then, I led her through a deep meditation in which she looked at her past and at how much she had accomplished in life thus far. In doing so, she was able to see that she had functioned well in spite of being abused as a child. She didn't want to do anything to jeopardize her companionship now and she felt that she had to change her ways to ensure that. There was an unlocking of the issue that had been keeping her in a limited reality.

Listening to her own answers and asking herself some powerful questions, Sylvia was able to realize that she was trying to please her companion, who loved an impeccably clean home. Having had parents who divorced and seeing all the unpleasantness around her own custody was hard on her and it kept coming back to her.

It turned out that the way Sylvia worked was by splattering bright paint with energy and enthusiasm without any worry of making a mess in her space. Now that her studio was in her house, she felt locked into the role of trying to keep it clean. This was crippling her and restraining her expression. We took the remaining time to itemize the expectations she held for herself in her marriage and her career and she sketched out her action steps for creating a healthy distance between the two. She was finally embracing her new reality.

Sylvia felt a great deal of responsibility about spending money on a separate studio space away from home. But it was clear to her that she didn't have to keep her studio in her home. We then took that opportunity to role-play Sylvia speaking to her partner about the new investment she was about to make, an especially difficult conversation after they had spent so much on the home. At first, she shut down. We tried it again and she was able to persevere. She told me what she wanted to say and then firmly but politely pushed back against the feelings of guilt she was experiencing.

By the following week, Sylvia had found and leased her new workspace. There was hope in her being and she was excited to prime the big canvas, her final piece for her upcoming exhibition. Sylvia finished her creative project and not only did she experience a lot of success with the exhibition, but she also found that she was not limited to only the "safest" choices. She was not restrained by the limitations and fears of her mind.

Three Tips for Creatives

1. Write to the prompt "How have I defined my creative reality?"
2. What are the chances that when you are not able to complete a creative project, it is because you are trying to protect yourself?
3. What is the one thing that is in your way?

Three Tips for Coaches

1. When you work with clients, keep in mind the possibility that exactly one thing may be stopping them from completing their work.
2. Explore that possibility with clients by asking, "Do you think it's possible that there is one thing in the way of you finishing?"
3. If a client does identify that one thing, invite them to next identify the actions steps necessary to deal with that "one thing."

About the Author

Pragati Chaudhry holds a degree in fine arts (MFA) and in teaching fine arts (MST) and loves leading people to a space where they stop creating from a place of struggle and start reclaiming their true creative power. She has had the privilege of working with extraordinary people from all around the world who followed their calling to connect with their creative alchemy. Trained as a creativity coach and as a life coach and having studied trauma-informed expressive arts therapy, she offers coaching and workshops for deep transformation through art and writing.

Journaling for Completion

40

Lynda Monk

There are many things that can support us to complete our creative work. Among them is our ability to know ourselves and our own unique ways of working toward and meeting the realities of completion and success in our lives.

One of my favorite tools for self-awareness is journaling. I also use it as a true companion practice to support me in my creative pursuits. There are many ways journaling helps my creative work and it can help you and your self-expressive work too.

Journaling can support you in your creative work by helping you do the following:

- Get focused, grounded and centered
- Set priorities and be clear about what matters most
- Brainstorm creative ideas and discover new projects
- Sift through options and choices and make decisions about your creative projects
- Capture fresh ideas for possible new projects
- Gather raw material that might end up being used in another form. For example, I often mine my journals for moments, memories, scenes and, dialogue to inform my memoir project.

Journaling can help you complete creative work by supporting you to identify and process emotional and mindset obstacles to completion so you can overcome them.

DOI: 10.4324/9781003351344-40

Five Common Obstacles to Completing Creative Work and Journal Prompts to Explore and Overcome Them

These journaling prompts can deepen your self-awareness and bring new insights that can support you and the completion of your creative work. Try to bring full self-compassion and nonjudgmental presence forward as you write and reflect. Emotions such as shame, guilt and feeling badly *do not* support creative self-expression. Self-compassion, self-kindness, curiosity and self-love open us to our greatest potential and help us complete the things we want to complete in our lives. I invite you to keep these virtues present as you reflect on common obstacles any of us might face when we strive to complete our creative work.

Obstacle #1 – Procrastination

Procrastination might very well be the number one obstacle to getting creative work completed. I recently participated in a Heal + Create Writer's Retreat and Lauren Sapala was one of the inspiring speakers at this event. Her topic was "Healing from Procrastination and Perfectionism: How Trauma Blocks Writers." She said that procrastination happens more often and readily for people who were raised to put other peoples' needs before their own. That really resonated with me. It has me thinking a lot more broadly about the complexities of both procrastination and perfectionism, which often live together.

Journaling Prompts for Exploring Procrastination

- What is one thing you have been putting off?
- Why do you think you keep putting it off – procrastinating, avoiding it, making other things more important?
- What is one step you can take to start working on it?
- What will get in the way of you taking that one step?
- How will you feel if you take that step?
- How do you want to celebrate when you have taken this step forward with completing your creative work? Celebrating your milestones can support your progress!

Obstacle #2 – Dealing With Distractions

Getting distracted is a normal part of the creative process and a normal part of life. Sure, some people can focus better than others. Some people have really worked hard to put strategies in place to help them focus and minimize distractions. For example, my friend Emma sets a timer and works on one task for a certain amount of time. While there are many other things calling for her attention, she minimizes distractions for set periods of time and she gets *a lot* of things done. If you find that you keep getting distracted, here are some journal prompts that might help you explore what is getting in the way or what is causing distractions so that you can overcome them.

Journaling Prompts for Dealing With Distractions

- What keeps pulling you away? For example, is it other people, the competing needs and priorities in your life, avoidance, or your dog walking across the room?
- What distracts you the most?
- What helps you minimize distractions? For example, turning off the notifications on your phone.
- What is at stake if you don't deal with distractions?
- How will letting distractions pull you away or interrupt you possibly sabotage or prevent you from getting your creative project completed?

Taking a moment to pause and reflect on where distractions are taking you or what they are preventing in your life can be a valuable step in helping you overcome them.

Obstacle #3 – Having Trouble Saying No

Being able to say no to some things allows you to say yes to other things. For example, we invited many creativity coaches and colleagues to be part of this book. Many of them said yes and we are grateful for their voices and wisdom in this book. Some individuals said no as they were prioritizing other projects, including things like focusing on promotion for their new memoir coming out, growing current creative offerings and so forth.

When I mentioned this project to one of my colleagues, Lucia Capacchione, who is the author of many books and knows how to get things done, she responded to me with an email that read:

> Saying no is so crucial to the creative process, especially completion. I cannot think of a better topic to focus on. I find that the women I work with have an especially hard time saying no to others and yes to themselves and their own projects. It takes a long time to learn and requires the support of others who have walked the path.

Journaling Prompts for Saying No

The word *no* is an important part of assertive communication and setting boundaries. Without it, we would say yes to everything and risk becoming overwhelmed and burned out.

- How easy is it for you to say no to the requests of others?
- How hard is it for you to say no?
- When have you said no to something so that you could say yes to working on and completing your creative work?
- How did that feel?
- When you witness other people say no and set limits with their time so they can prioritize their creative work, how do you feel about them? Do you admire them? Resent them? Wish you could do that too? Just get curious about this. We can learn a lot about our own relationship to the word *no* by witnessing how we feel about other peoples' nos.

Obstacle #4 – Not Having Clear Goals and Priorities

I was born under the sign of Virgo and I'm a natural goal setter. I have annual, quarterly, monthly, weekly and daily goals written down and prioritized. I review my goals regularly, mark them as complete and reschedule ones I didn't get to yet to be done on the path ahead. I often have more goals and tasks on my list than I can possibly get done in the time I allow. I have to constantly prioritize to ensure the most important things are what I am doing next. I have learned that goal setting and prioritizing are key skills and tasks required to get projects done. I don't get every creative project finished, mostly because I am more ambitious and optimistic with my goals and less realistic with how much time tasks will actually take to complete. Nonetheless, I get *a lot* of things completed each and every day. Having clear goals and priorities combined with taking daily actions toward them adds up to a significant body of creative work completed over time.

Journaling Prompts for Gaining Clarity and Setting Priorities

- How do you feel about goal setting when it comes to your creative work?
- Do you have SMART (specific, measurable, action-oriented, realistic and time limited) goals?
- What are your priorities this week that will help you reach your goals?
- How do these priorities align with your big goals and creative dreams?
- What action steps must you take to reach your goals?
- What do you need to *start* doing or *stop* doing to achieve your goals and complete your creative work?

For example, I have recently stopped spending time on Facebook, with the exception of a journaling group I run, to make more time for working on my adoptee memoir. While I only spent a few minutes a day here and there on Facebook, it all added up and that time can be reallocated to a higher-value activity that will help me complete my memoir project.

Obstacle #5 – Being Impatient

Yes, it's true – we want to engage momentum with our creative projects and pursuits. In fact, I think it is important to contribute real time to our creative projects each and every day to maintain our focus, intention and commitment to completion. And it is important to be patient.

Patience takes the pressure off of us while not letting us off the hook for keeping our commitments to ourselves. Patience and trust live close together. We have to trust ourselves that we can get things done; we need to trust that our creative self-expression is a valuable part of making meaning in our lives. We need to trust that even if things are going slower than we want them to, patience is part of progress. It is also part of letting ourselves rest and not constantly be pushing. Our creativity needs time and space, breathing space . . . and we need the same.

Journaling Prompts to Cultivate Patience

- What helps you be easy on yourself?
- When do you find yourself feeling impatient?
- What does patience feel like to you?
- How do you know when you are being patient?
- What value does patience have, or could it have, as you complete your creative work?

For example, I often feel impatient that my adoptee memoir is not written yet, that it is not complete. But I have grown to appreciate that I am still living the unfolding of the story, that there were important situations I had to go through and more parts of the story that had to reveal themselves to me. For example, I recently learned the identity of my biological father's family. I am still narrowing down who my biological dad is because he is one of five brothers, only two of whom are still alive. In any case, I will have half siblings as all these men had other children. Ultimately, I have grown to believe that more of life and my experience as an adoptee, a daughter and a mother had to be experienced so that I could tell the story my memoir is meant to tell. I have to trust this and have patience with myself as a writer and with the writing process itself.

Completing Makes a Difference

As a coach, I have worked with hundreds of clients over the years. I have regularly witnessed that when someone can reflect on, address and overcome, or at least minimize, some of these common obstacles and experiences with creative work, they are much more likely to be successful with completion and the realization of creative dreams.

Completing any creative project successfully takes thought, planning, conscious action and devotion. Even when we have clear goals and a plan and take consistent action, there may be many challenges and obstacles that come up along the way. We cannot predict these when we first start our projects. Journaling about our thoughts and feelings along the creative path helps us to gain clarity, as well as the necessary inspiration and motivation from within to support us to successfully complete and celebrate our creative work.

I believe we are living in what creativity coach and artist Laura Hollick, founder of Soul Art Studio, describes as the Age of the Artist. She says that we are living in transformative times where the old ways of living and being are changing, falling away and creatives are needed, called upon to literally help create this next evolution in our human history. Our world needs its artists, creatives, innovators, intuitives, resisters and revolutionaries. . . . Our world needs *you and your completed work.*

Three Tips for Creatives

1. Keep a regular journal to support the emotional and psychological journey of overcoming any obstacles to completing your creative work.
2. Let yourself project how you will feel when your creative goal is accomplished even before you have it completed. For example, I might say to myself, "I am so happy and grateful now that my adoptee memoir has been published and is getting rave reviews."
3. Use affirmations for completion. Create affirmations or use the ones that follow. Write them down and keep them where you can see them. Say them to yourself to keep your positive "completion" mindset activated.

   - "I am living my purposes through completing."
   - "I have greater freedom as a person who completes things."
   - "Completion is a gift I give to the world."
   - "I am in my integrity when I finish what I say I'm going to do."
   - "I create a meaningful life through completions."
   - "I honor myself through completing."

Three Tips for Coaches

1. Most importantly, complete the things you set out to complete. Lead completion by example! Keep your own journal for writing about your thoughts, feelings and creative projects. Let journaling help you overcome obstacles to completion by going to the page to deal with what gets in the way.

2. Support your clients to gain clarity about *why* they are doing their creative project – having a strong *why* helps clients do what it takes to complete what matters most to them. Know your own *why* as a coach. Why do *you* do what you do? This makes a great journaling prompt.

3. At the end of every group coaching program I facilitate, in our closing circle when each participant offers final comments about their experience, I invite them to say, "I am complete." Acknowledging and bringing the energy of completion into our coaching helps our clients bring the felt sense of completion into their own creative work and lives.

I am complete.

 ## About the Author

Lynda Monk, MSW, RSW, CPCC is the director of the International Association for Journal Writing. She is the co-author and co-editor of four books on writing, journaling and creativity. The most recent publication, co-edited with Eric Maisel, is *The Great Book of Journaling: How Journal Writing Can Support a Life of Wellness, Creativity, Meaning and Purpose.* Lynda regularly writes, teaches and speaks about the healing and transformational power of writing. She loves leading and growing the IAJW.org, which is an inspirational and educational community for journal writers worldwide. You can sign-up to receive her weekly *Journaling Museletter* and get a free journaling gift at http://iajw.org/journalwriting.

Co-Editor's Conclusion

12 Tips for Completing Your Creative Projects

Eric Maisel

The following are twelve tips for completing your creative projects. Give them a try!

1. Hold the Intention to Complete Your Creative Projects

I hope that the discussion in this book has made it clear why many creatives who suppose that they want to complete their creative projects are actually harboring more reasons for leaving their work unfinished than reasons for completing their work. You, too, may have many reasons for wanting to leave your creative projects unfinished. One counter to all those reasons is a strong intention to finish the work you start. With each new project, say, "I intend to finish this!" Naturally, some projects will deserve to be abandoned and some will prove too difficult to complete. Those hard realities, however, are not reasons to hold anything less than an abiding desire to complete what you start.

2. Recognize That Completing Your Creative Projects Is a Challenge in Its Own Right

Even if you want to complete your creative projects, even if you are manifesting no self-sabotaging energy or negative thoughts, completing them may remain a real challenge. Making something good isn't easy and making

DOI: 10.4324/9781003351344-41

something great is that much harder. If creating an excellent thing were easy, we would see many more masterworks. But completing even quite ordinary creative work is hard in its own right: getting to the end of your novel, your mural, or your symphony isn't easy, whether it is great or ordinary or even less than good. Accept this reality and counter it with effort and energy.

3. Get Clear on Why You Aren't Completing Your Creative Projects

If you're in the habit of not completing your creative projects, figure out why. There may be one persistent reason, there may be several persistent reasons, or each project may be its own situation. Maybe self-doubt always enters the equation. Maybe it's a fear or loathing of the marketplace. Maybe it's a lack of organization and a chaotic way of being that, as the work grows, causes you to throw up your hands and surrender to the chaos and disorganization. Maybe it's last-minute self-censorship and an inchoate desire to hide. Maybe the work is regularly poorly constructed and fails to meet your own standards. The possible reasons are legion. It is your job to figure out what's going on and what's keeping you from completing projects.

4. Use Your Existential Intelligence as an Aid in Completing

Use your existential intelligence and your native ability to think about meaning and life purpose as aids in helping you complete your creative projects. When you get clear that finishing your creative work provides you with the psychological experience of meaning and meets your life purpose intentions, you have more reasons for completing than just making beautiful things or making things that sell. By putting completing your creative projects in the category of life purpose choice, you provide yourself with more motivational energy to finish and deeper reasons for finishing.

5. Create a Completion Checklist

Devise a way of creating a punch list that helps you check off tasks. If, for example, you are doing something as complicated as making an independent film, you are obliged to work from such lists if you are to keep all the myriad details straight and the enterprise on schedule. Even if you are doing something ostensibly less complicated, like writing a song, you might still contrive a way of creating and using a completion checklist, maybe including such items as lyrics, melody, bridge, tempo change and resolution. A completion checklist may not be appropriate for your current creative project – but it may be. Give this idea some thought!

6. Practice Anxiety Management

Our doubts, worries and nerves prevent us from getting finished. Anxiety threads its way through the creative process and anxiety is most present as we try to complete our work. Learn one or several anxiety management techniques, like a deep breathing or relaxation technique, to help you reduce your experience of anxiety, approach your nearly finished work and stay put as you endeavor to finish it.

7. Practice Right Thinking

Get and keep a grip on your mind. Nothing does a better job of getting in the way of you completing your creative projects than the thoughts you think that don't serve you. Thinking a thought as innocuous as "I'm very busy today" or "I don't have that much energy" can do a perfect job of keeping you from tackling your current creative project. Remember the simple three-step process for dealing with thoughts that don't serve you: hear what you are thinking, actively dispute any thought that isn't serving you and substitute a more useful and affirmative thought for the thought you just disputed. Pay attention to this every day!

8. If You Do Put a Project Aside, Create a Plan for Returning

You may have excellent reasons for putting a creative project aside for the time being. But even if you have excellent reasons for putting it aside, you will want to create a plan and/or a schedule for getting back to it. The plan might be as simple as "As soon as I return from China, I will get back to my novel" or it may be more elaborate and take many eventualities and contingencies into account. Imagine the sort of plan you'd want to create to return to your incomplete suite of paintings that are being held up because your arthritis is acting up, because you're waiting for certain special pigments to arrive, because the narrative thread of several of the paintings is eluding you and because you're in negotiations with a gallery for a solo show. Mightn't this set of circumstances benefit from a plan?

9. Get Strategic Help

You're trying to finish up your independent film documentary, but a handful of tasks stand between you and completion. Some of them are technical and require new learning; some are artistic but not in areas that you know well. You might be able to gain the technical expertise, but do spending the time on that and dealing with the stress of a steep learning curve outweigh the expense of hiring someone? You might be able to master the artistic part, but is learning to score your film the best use of your time, or might it not be better to see if there are low-cost or free film scorers available who might help you? Part of us wants to do everything ourselves and retain complete control, but that stance can stop us in our tracks when we face tasks that we do not know how to handle.

10. Repeat What's Worked

Say that you write novels and you've had the following experiences. Each time you've had a clear picture in your mind about how a given novel ends, you've successfully completed that novel. For some reason – on a whim almost – you decided that with your current novel, you will only know how it ends "when you got there." But you haven't been able to get there and you've been stalled now for months. It's your decision whether to adamantly and stubbornly stick to your whimsical decision or do what previously worked. Very often, we get an odd idea in our head – say, the odd idea that it would be "cheating" to know how our novel ends – and get ourselves stuck for absolutely no good reason. If something has worked for you in the past, please consider doing it again. And, by the same token, avoid doing what hasn't worked!

11. Visualize Completion and Success

It pays to picture success. If you're writing a symphony, get a clear picture in mind of an orchestra playing it. If you're painting a suite of paintings, visualize them on the walls of an upscale gallery. If you're working on a screenplay, enjoy the prospect of a Hollywood opening night, red carpet and all. Likewise, visualize abundance as your body of work grows: picture your current novel joining other novels of yours on a bookcase shelf, your current CD joining other CDs of yours in a handsome CD case. Most importantly, visualize you completing your current project: see yourself putting that last period on your manuscript and, with a smile of pride on your face, getting up from your computer. Picture both, success and completion!

12. Show Up

Virtually every question connected to completing your creative project is answered by the act of showing up. It may not be answered in one day; on a given day, you may sit there, paralyzed and defeated, as nothing comes to you. On a given day, you may go backward or sideways. But if you show up again the next day and the next day and the next day, the ice is likely to thaw, the horizon is likely to become visible and real progress is the likely outcome. No alcoholic is told, "You only need to go to one AA meeting. That's plenty!" Nor should any creative imagine that showing up to his work only occasionally is sufficient. Institute a regular practice; do the work and while completing your creative projects may not be guaranteed as a result, you can take it to the bank that you will have dramatically upped your odds of success.

About Eric Maisel

Eric Maisel is the author of 50+ books. His recent books include *Why Smart Teens Hurt*, *Redesign Your Mind* and *The Power of Daily Practice*. Among his other books are *Coaching the Artist Within*, *Fearless Creating*, *Rethinking Depression* and *The Van Gogh Blues*. Dr. Maisel writes the *Rethinking Mental Health* blog for *Psychology Today*, with 3,000,000+ views and is the creator and lead editor for the Ethics International Press Critical Psychology and Critical Series.

A retired family therapist and active creativity coach, Dr. Maisel's forthcoming books include *The Coach's Way* (New World Library) and *Deconstructing ADHD* (Ethics International Press). Dr. Maisel provides workshops, webinars and keynotes nationally and internationally; trains creativity coaches; and facilitates support groups for writers. You can visit him at www.ericmaisel. com and contact him at ericmaisel@hotmail.com.

About Lynda Monk

Lynda Monk, MSW, RSW, CPCC is a registered social worker, a certified life coach and the director of the International Association for Journal Writing – IAJW.org. She leads a global creative community especially for journal writers with members from countries around the world. Lynda is co-editor, with Eric Maisel, of two books: *Transformational Journaling for Coaches, Therapists and Clients: A Complete Guide to the Benefits of Personal Writing* and *The Great Book of Journaling: How Journal Writing Can Support a Life of Wellness, Creativity, Meaning and Purpose.* She is the co-author of *Writing Alone Together: Journaling in a Circle of Women for Creativity, Compassion and Connection.* She developed *Life Source Writing: A 5-Step Journaling Method for Self-Discovery, Self-Care, Wellness and Creativity.* Lynda regularly teaches, writes and speaks on the healing and transformational power of journaling and expressive writing. She is currently writing her adoptee memoir, a labor of love that she is committed to completing. Lynda lives with her family on Salt Spring Island, British Columbia, Canada, where she tries her best to write every day.

Index

Page numbers in *italic* indicate a figure and page numbers in **bold** indicate a table on the corresponding page

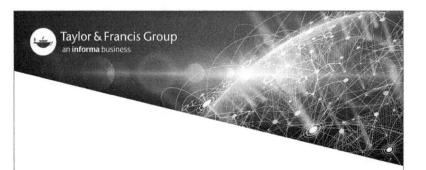